Back to Reform

Back to Reform

*Values, Markets, and
the Health Care System*

Charles J. Dougherty

New York   Oxford
OXFORD UNIVERSITY PRESS
1996

Oxford University Press

Oxford   New York
Athens   Auckland   Bangkok   Bombay
Calcutta   Cape Town   Dar es Salaam   Delhi
Florence   Hong Kong   Istanbul   Karachi
Kuala Lumpur   Madras   Madrid   Melbourne
Mexico City   Nairobi   Paris   Singapore
Taipei   Tokyo   Toronto

and associated companies in
Berlin   Ibadan

Library of Congress Cataloging-in-Publication Data
Dougherty, Charles J., 1949–
Back to reform : values, markets, and the health
care system / Charles J. Dougherty.
p.   cm.   Includes index.
ISBN 0-19-510397-1
1. Health care reform—Moral and ethical
aspects—United States.
I. Title.
RA395.A3D676   1996
362.1'0973—dc20   95-50069

9 8 7 6 5 4 3 2 1

Printed in the United States of America
on acid-free paper

To my parents,
who taught me a great deal about values
but never so much as when health
and health care failed them.

Preface

There is an anecdote that seems increasingly apt as the health care system changes under the enormous pressure of market forces. The story goes that the pilot of a commercial airliner traveling through a storm announces to the passengers that he has good news and bad news. The bad news, he reports, is that there has been an electrical problem in the cockpit that has caused all the plane's directional equipment to malfunction. Since the storm prohibits determining bearings by sight, "We don't know which way we're going." When the passengers begin to panic, the pilot returns to remind them that there is also good news: "We're making great time!"

In the fall of 1993, it seemed that the health care system was headed for a thorough overhaul, guided by the Clinton administration's plan to achieve universal coverage and contain costs by way of managed competition. Within less than a year, however, it became clear that federally directed health care reform would not occur, at least not in the foreseeable future.

Failure in Washington did not mean the health care system would remain unchanged. On the contrary, powerful market forces led by a payer rebellion are changing the health care system in fundamental ways and with a rapidity few could have anticipated. All care is now managed care in one form or other. Capitation is sweeping fee-for-service aside. Indemnity insurers are organizing health maintenance organizations, or HMOs. Doctors are becoming employees. Specialties are being overshadowed by primary care. Hospitals are now cost centers, not revenue generators. Inpatient census and length of stay continue to plummet. Delivery networks and corporate alliances are forming everywhere, integrating services vertically (hospital–physician group–home health care) and horizontally (hospital–hospital). Indeed, "We're making great time!"

Like the plane in the anecdote, however, change in the health care system has no overall sense of direction. Cost containment is the main theme, as many of these changes are provoked by employer and insurer refusals to absorb continued cost increases. Yet there are no global curbs on costs; they still rise faster than the consumer price index. Access problems continue to worsen, and the new financial parsimony has raised concerns about the quality of care.

There is rapid health care change, but change is not inherently positive. The system still needs reform. Health care reform requires improvement, not only change but change in the right direction. To appraise change, to determine where it amounts to reform and where it does not, an overall sense of direction is needed. In the final analysis, moral values provide that sense of direction. They are the ultimate benchmarks for measuring health care reform.

The goal of this book is to begin a conversation on the moral values that should direct change in the health care system. It is an attempt to retrieve the directional equipment needed to chart a new course back to health care reform.

The overall strategy is to identify key moral values, display their roots and general structures, and apply them to the health care system with the purpose of criticizing current trends and providing a normative framework for reform. The values themselves are identified from reflection on a shared world of moral concepts that recur in health care and health care ethics contexts: human dignity, caring, protection of the least well off, the common good, cost containment, responsibility, and excellence. There is no pretense that these are the only moral values at stake in the health care system, but these are important moral values and they are at stake. These familiar if elusive values probably have multiple roots. Two of the deeper, more significant roots are explored here: the Judeo-Christian religious tradition and the Enlightenment secular tradition. The structure frequently revealed within these values is oppositional: individual rights versus the common good, markets versus mission, freedom versus regulation, and determinism versus free will. The application of values to the health care system is broadly Aristotlean. Virtue is sought by holding opposing tendencies in creative tension and favoring the least stressed tendency to achieve greater balance.

Significant failures and imbalances exist in the present health care system in the United States. Awareness of this fact motivated recent efforts for health care reform. Although those efforts collapsed, the failures and imbalances in the system remain. No doubt, the rapid and in some ways revolutionary market changes sweeping through the system will bring some improvements; but it is equally clear that they will also exacerbate some of the system's failures and exaggerate some of its imbalances. Moreover, market changes tend as a rule to be unconscious of moral values—sometimes supportive, sometimes inimical, generally unaware. Reflection on moral values is therefore critical for two reasons: to curb the worst excesses of the directionless change that is reshaping the system and, most importantly, to set the stage for renewed efforts to reform the system consciously. The first lesson of reflection on these values is that health care reform remains a moral imperative.

Contents

Back to Reform

1

The Health Care System

Change and Reform

At the end of the twentieth century, the American health care system is beset by continued access problems, escalating costs, and concerns about quality. These problems have provoked a variety of government-initiated attempts at reform, attempts that have failed or have been only marginally successful. The defeat of the Clinton plan virtually assures that there will be no large-scale federal health care reform effort in the near future. States have had some minor successes but face limited resources and authority. Reform of the system is beyond their capacities.

Nevertheless, tremendous changes are occurring throughout the health care system.[1] Employers and insurers (the same entity in the case of most large employers) have rebelled against constant cost increases. They have united in communities across the nation to force providers to offer discounts and to reconstruct local delivery systems to cut costs. These marketplace pressures are forcing hospitals to downsize as rates of hospitalization and lengths of stay are pushed lower. Care is managed with an eye toward greater efficiency. Capitation is replacing fee-for-service throughout the system. New delivery networks are forming that combine hospitals, doctors, and payers and that create a vertical integration of services from clinics to home health care to hospice. Hospitals and health systems are merging and forming corporate alliances that create horizontal integration in local communities and regions. The rise of delivery networks and the decline of the previously central role of hospitals have meant a renewed demand for primary care providers and a consequent collapse of demand for specialists. The movement toward group practice of medicine has accelerated, and many groups and individual doctors have sold their practices to networks and become employees. Medicaid programs across the nation are adopting managed-care techniques and beginning to contract with single providers and to pay by capitation. Consumers and patients have fewer choices and more copayments. These and other market adjustments will continue to produce dramatic changes in the system into the foreseeable future.

The sweeping political changes begun by the congressional elections in the fall of 1994 have accelerated these market-driven forces. The role of government in health care has been reduced, and federal money and influence have been transferred to state and local levels. This change in political philosophy— less government, not more—makes federally led health care reform improbable in the foreseeable future. Major change in the health care system is now driven by market reforms, by the invisible yet powerful hand of the marketplace.

The demand for reform, however, intends not simply a different health care system, but a better one. Whether the changes sweeping the system will actually improve it is an open question that can be addressed in several ways. Health outcome is one standard. Improvements sufficient to be called *reform* must be marked by improved health statistics for the nation as a whole, and especially for groups who have suffered from higher rates of morbidity and mortality. Reform can also be assessed with respect to economic performance. An improved system would have to be financially leaner and have sustainable rates of growth. Reform can also be measured in political terms. A reformed system would be more politically acceptable, enjoying wide support among citizens and providers.

Because health care deals so directly with so many deeply important matters—life, quality of life, vulnerability, caring, dying, death, and so on—there is one other measure of reform that must be appraised. There must be an ethical assessment of whether a changed system better embodies the moral values of Americans.[2] Is the system improved with respect to the most important values attached to health care?

This question might be approached descriptively, perhaps by using survey instruments that poll the public about its values and assess to what extent the public finds these values embodied in the health care system. Whereas a descriptive approach like this may make an important contribution to a general ethical assessment, it is not always the most appropriate methodology when dealing with values, and it is not the approach adopted here. The inherent complexity of moral values often defeats even the most determined and subtle descriptive analyses. More importantly, values are norms. They state or describe what *ought* to be, not what is. This aspect of values must be captured directly, in their own realities as values. For these reasons, ethical assessment of reform must include a normative appraisal of the values at stake in health care.

Theoretically, there is a large chasm between factual description and normative prescription, between the "is" and the "ought" of experience. A report about what people believe they ought to do—smokers agreeing that they ought to stop smoking, for example—may create little normative impact. A strongly motivated norm, for example, that "sin taxes" should pay for universal health insurance coverage, may have little basis in fact.[3] More important, the fact that many Americans espouse a moral value does not of itself make that moral value valid. Precisely what does—or should—confer such validity is one of the deepest and most difficult issues in ethical theory; but it is clear that the facts of what a majority holds at any one time, even as a tradition held across generations, do not suffice to establish ethical validity. They do, however, create an important moral reality, a given mix of facts and values, that can provide a platform for critical reflection, even if the rules for criticism are themselves underdetermined.

Despite these theoretical difficulties, there are facts and there are values. The former constitute reality as we imagine it, separate from our aspirations and fears; the latter are the realities of our aspirations and fears. The real world of daily life is experienced as a web of interlinked facts and values. There is no world of facts without values, since values themselves (impartiality, for example) are required for facts. There is no world of values without facts, since having a value is itself a fact. To embark on a normative inquiry, however, requires that (some) values be isolated and analyzed separate from (some) facts to some extent, though never completely. Because such critical reflection cannot pretend to absolute ethical validity or even to complete isolation of all the relevant facts and values, it requires a method that is open-ended, exploratory, and subject to self-correction.

Such a method is philosophical. It is a self-reflective inquiry proceeding not from a detached scientific standpoint, but from within the values themselves. As such, it can easily devolve into dogmatism or autobiography, representing merely the ideas and experiences of the author. There is only one strategy for dealing with this potential: adoption of a conversational intent at the outset. This book does not pretend to be *the* statement of the values at stake in a changing health care system. The perspective developed here is admittedly a point of view from within the values themselves. If it is to be more than that, if it is to achieve wider intersubjective validity, it must be offered as a moment in a larger national conversation in which many and diverse voices are invited to share other perspectives, fill in omissions, and correct misinterpretations. This book proposes to make a contribution to that conversation.

Access Problems

To set the stage for an explicitly ethical analysis, some of the main problem areas in the health care system must be identified. Articulation of these problems need not be exhaustive, since the direct aim is ethical analysis of values. Nonetheless, there must be a common understanding of the general character of the problems in the system that have provoked the need for reform.

The most longstanding problem in the system that has generated energy for reform is the problem of access. In 1995, approximately forty million Americans had no health insurance coverage.[4] These people are not eligible for Medicare or Medicaid and do not have any private insurance coverage. They are literally uncovered and would have to pay out of pocket in the event health care were needed. Most are at or near the bottom of the socioeconomic scale and would be financially incapable of paying directly the costs of any serious health care intervention. Recent reform efforts intended to eliminate this problem by achieving universal coverage, but they failed. The number of uninsured peoples continues to increase, and the efforts toward incremental reform are unlikely to reverse this trend. The fact remains that despite considerable political agreement on the goal of universal coverage, millions of Americans remain without health insurance coverage and are likely to be so into the foreseeable future.[5]

Some have dismissed the significance of this number by pointing out, correctly, that the figure of forty million uninsured represents a "snapshot" in time and that a more dynamic picture would show that over time many of these uninsured people will obtain coverage.[6] In the mid-1980s, for example, half of all periods without health insurance ended within six months. This objection, however, which is designed to minimize the problem as merely transitional, proves too much. First, it shows that more than half of the periods without health insurance last longer than six months. In fact, about twenty-eight percent of all uninsured spells last more than a year; from fifteen to eighteen percent last more than two years. Second, it shows that the numbers of Americans without insurance for some time in any given period must be very large because if some twenty million are gaining insurance every six months and the figure of forty million is an accurate snapshot at any time, then another twenty million must be losing health insurance every six months. The best guess in 1992 was that one of every four nonelderly Americans was without health insurance sometime during the year. Finally, the optimistic view that being without health insurance is only a temporary inconvenience for some Americans overlooks the logic of health insurance. Regardless of the fact that a person or family may become covered in the future, even the near future, if they are uninsured at the time medical treatment is needed, there is no coverage for that treatment. Each uninsured moment is a risk, a real insecurity for both individuals and families. More importantly, if a serious health condition is treated or diagnosed during a period when there is no insurance, however long or short the period, that health condition may be excluded from future insurance coverage as a preexisting illness, creating devastating financial and medical problems for many Americans, especially for children and young adults.

It is true that some of those without health care coverage are young people at low risk for health problems who choose to remain without coverage because the cost of insurance is high and their perceived need for health care is low, but even the young and the healthy can find themselves in need of health care. Aside from the statistically small numbers of cancers, heart disease, and strokes that strike some young and apparently healthy people each year, this group is especially subject to automobile accidents, injuries at work and play, drug and alcohol abuse, and all the health effects of domestic and street violence. Young, healthy women also have most of the nation's babies. When uninsured, they are less likely to have adequate prenatal care.

Many of the uninsured are not young, healthy adults; they are Americans of all ages below age sixty-five. A third are children. The vast majority live in households headed by someone working full-time, someone whose fringe benefits do not include health insurance. Typically, these workers are employed by small businesses such as fast-food chains, small construction companies, laundries, retail outlets, and the like. Many are acutely aware of their lack of coverage but, because their earnings are low, cannot afford to pay the high premiums involved.

As mentioned, other Americans have exclusions in their health insurance that deny coverage for treatments related to conditions that preexisted initiation of their present coverage.[7] For some, this means the cost of the care they are most likely to need is not insured. Because portability of health insurance is not guaranteed throughout the system, others face "job-lock," the fear that a change in employment will jeopardize all or part of their family's health insurance coverage because of preexisting illnesses.[8] Others remain among the "uninsurable," those individuals and families whose experience of catastrophic health care illness and associated costs make them too high a risk for private insurance carriers.

Many uninsured Americans are able to access health care, but their care is likely to be provided in hospital emergency rooms, where it is not likely to be timely, comprehensive, or personal. The emergency room is also one of the most expensive providers in the entire health care system. The cost of this uncompensated, expensive care is shifted by hospitals to other patients and their payers, especially to private insurers after Medicare and Medicaid began systematically underpaying hospital charges in the mid-1980s.[9] Moreover, studies over the last decade have consistently shown that the financial barriers to health care faced by the uninsured jeopardize their health and cause preventable deaths.[10]

Untold numbers of Americans are turned away or discouraged from accessing health care.[11] Many simply delay or refuse to seek needed health care, with the predictable consequences for their health. Thus, the lack of universal and portable health insurance creates substantial access problems for large numbers of Americans. In 1993, for example, thirty-four percent of the uninsured reported that they did not receive needed care, and seventy-one percent postponed needed care because of inability to pay for it.[12] As a group, uninsured adults make thirty-nine percent fewer ambulatory visits than insured adults and have thirty-three percent fewer hospital days per person; uninsured children make thirty percent fewer ambulatory visits and have nineteen percent fewer hospital days. The negative effect of the lack of insurance is even clearer when access is measured among adults and children in fair to poor health. Among these more medically needy Americans, uninsured adults make forty percent fewer ambulatory visits than their insured peers and have thirty-nine percent fewer hospital days; the rates for uninsured children with fair to poor health are forty-five percent fewer ambulatory visits and fifty-one percent fewer hospital days.[13] These figures show marked, significant differences in access to care as the result of insurance status.

Other access problems beset the system, even for insured persons. The vast distances between providers in rural and frontier areas of the nation constitute a significant access barrier for many Americans. In the inner cities, many who have private insurance or who qualify for Medicare and Medicaid still face transportation difficulties and serious overcrowding in the hospitals that serve these communities. Moreover, one in six Medicaid beneficiaries reports that their coverage has been refused by a doctor or hospital, and about the same percent claim they have to rely on a hospital emergency room because they do not have a regular doctor.[14] This phenomenon is likely to increase as responsibility for Medicaid is increasingly turned over to the states. Many Americans from minority racial and ethnic groups also face barriers related to culture and language. There are also many noncitizens working in the United States who, fearing discovery and deportation, refuse to seek access to the health care system for help with bona fide health problems.

In spite of continued criticism on this score and market pressures against it, the health care system still displays a decided disposition toward acute-care interventions by doctors with subspecialty training. In many parts of the country, this disposition creates difficulties in accessing a primary care provider.[15] Subspecialty care, as important as it can be, tends by its very nature to be less holistic and therefore less personal. It also tends to slight prevention. Throughout the health care system, far too little money and effort is invested in advance of the context of need to keep individuals and communities healthy.

At the other end of the continuum of health care, there simply is no system of long-term care.[16] For most Americans, long-term custodial care for elderly or disabled family members means "spending down" household resources until the impoverishment requirements of Medicaid are reached. The growing numbers of very old Americans, patients with Alzheimer's disease and acquired immunodeficiency syndrome (AIDS)-related dementia, and survivors of trauma who need total care make this situation intolerable.

All the access issues above involve circumstances in which there is no or too little care in the face of real need. On the other hand, the American health care system also continues to provide too much treatment in other contexts, especially in treatment of the incompetent terminally ill, many of whom receive procedures they probably do not want and that only serve to prolong the dying process. There continue to be difficulties in determining the appropriate uses of life-preserving technology and in communicating this information effectively to patients and families.[17] Fears among both doctors and patients about the irrevocable character of choices to accept death continue to conspire to make death harder than it has to be for many Americans. Ironically, reluctance on the part of health care providers to allow patients to die, of the kind dramatized in the 1975 Karen Anne Quinlan case, for example, has been replaced in many instances by a reluctance of family members to accept the deaths of loved ones, in spite of doctors' assessments that continued struggle is futile. Even when doctors urge appropriate restraint in using extraordinary measures in cases of terminal illness—and doctors have improved significantly over the last generation in this regard—families too often demand that "everything" be done for (and to) their dying loved ones.

Costs

Rising costs continue to pose serious problems for the system. In fact, it is probably fair to say that recent efforts at health care reform would not have been mounted had those concerned about financial issues not joined forces with those concerned about access. Failure in these efforts to build consensus on a plan for universal coverage can be traced to the uneasy coalition of these two groups, especially to the reluctance of big business to accept a solution to its health care cost problems that involves a strong role for the federal government.

Another obvious dimension of the failed attempt at reform by the Clinton administration is the long-standing and significant mismatch between the value aspirations of most Americans for universal coverage combined with a reluctance to accept the tax increase necessary to pay for it. Polls since 1938 have shown a very high level of support for universal coverage, support that drops precipitously as the readiness to pay for it by increased taxation is assessed.[18] At the height of the debate over the Clinton plan, polls showed that an increase of only thirty dollars a month (or $360 annually) could not get majority support. Worse yet, a majority of Americans believed they would not gain from systemic reform, that reform would cost them more for what they already had, perhaps even taking away what they already had while costing them more.[19] Thus cost remains a central part of health care politics, as well it should.

In 1995 total spending on the health care system approaches one trillion dollars and could double by the year 2000.[20] In 1995 this amount represents about fifteen percent of the nation's gross domestic product (GDP); spending projected for the year 2000 would represent about twenty percent. The heart of the cost problem is not so much the number of dollars spent nor the percentage of the GDP it represents, staggering though they are. The heart of the matter and a genuine cause for alarm is the rate of growth in health care spending, which is especially clear when contemporary spending is compared with past spending. In many ways, the post-World War II period is the earliest reasonable point of comparison because it represents the beginning of contemporary health care in the United States. That period brought significant expansion of the hospital infrastructure and of medical school enrollment as well as dramatic new developments in surgery and pharmaceuticals. Spending for health care in 1950 was approximately five percent of the GDP. If twenty percent is reached by the year 2000, spending will have doubled twice in a 50-year period. Were this growth rate to continue for the next fifty years, by the mid-point of the twenty-first century, Americans would be devoting eighty percent of their GDP to health care. Obviously, this is an economically impossible scenario. No modern economy could devote so much of its economic effort and so much of the value of its goods and services to one activity. The conclusion is unavoidable: Even if costs continue to increase, the rate of increase itself must be reduced.

This dramatic increase in spending at the end of the twentieth century has taken its toll on various payers.[21] It has made a major contribution to the federal deficit and has created chaos in state budgets around the nation. It has

caused multiple personal and business bankruptcies. The international com-
petitiveness of American businesses has been compromised. There has been
a considerable increase in the amount of household income spent on
health care through increased taxes, higher insurance premiums, and new
copayments.

The list of candidates for the root cause of this cost explosion is long and
controverted.[22] Most agree that there is far too much capacity in the American hospital sector. Development and diffusion of new medical technology
and pharmaceuticals have been very expensive. Salaries of many who work
in the provider community have escalated, notably among specialty doctors,
hospital administrators, and insurance executives. Health insurance itself tends
to insulate providers and consumers from the true costs of health care interventions. Heightened fear of legal liability throughout the health care sector
has caused many new direct costs in legal fees, court costs, malpractice insurance, and risk managers. These direct costs are more than matched by the
untold indirect costs associated with defensive medicine, that is, the practice
of ordering more tests and documentation than necessary for quality health
care with the goal of avoiding or defending against malpractice suits.[23]

There has been little rational planning in the system, and expensive medical technologies have been duplicated needlessly in many American communities. Spending on administration of health care and on financial management
has increased dramatically.[24] New costs in this area include, ironically, those
associated with efforts to contain costs. Multiple attempts have been made
to micromanage the financial behavior of providers through preadmission
certification of hospitalization, utilization review, and similar procedures.
Many new costs are associated with increased competition in the health care
arena: advertising and other marketing costs, investment for strategic posi-
tioning against competitors, acquisitions of hospitals and doctors' practices,
and so on.

The ravages of human immunodeficiency virus (HIV), the explosion of gang
violence, and the persistence of large pockets of grinding poverty and despair
have all added to the health care account. Americans are living longer and
therefore experiencing more health care needs in their advanced ages. Overall, public expectations from health care have increased dramatically, including the expectation that every disease has a cure and that life can be lived
with vigor and enjoyment well past the biblical "three score and ten." As more
Americans are living longer, costs in the Medicare program have far exceeded
original projections from the mid-1960s and even the more experience-based
projections of the 1980s. Program costs exceeded $100 billion in 1985 and
reached about $150 billion in 1995. A Congressional Budget Office study
projects costs of $400 billion by the year 2004.[25] The Medicaid population
has expanded, in part because of the persistence of poverty, in part because

of federal mandates.[26] At the same time, the federal government has spent lavishly on tax shelters provided to corporations and individuals for private health insurance since the end of World War II.[27]

Recent private sector efforts to contain costs hold some promise of improvement in some of these areas. Nonetheless, the struggle to contain costs will be a central part of the challenge of health care reform well into the foreseeable future.

Quality

The last general category of problems triggering the need for systemic reform centers around quality, a clear strength of the system in the last half of the twentieth century. High standards of quality have been achieved and maintained throughout the U.S. hospital system, in doctors' offices, and at other sites of care. Much of this positive track record is attributable to the generally high quality of educational programs for health care professionals, graduate medical training for doctors, and the rigors of accreditation and licensing processes throughout the system.[28] It is this noteworthy success that is likely on the minds of those who assert that the United States has the best health care system in the world. In many respects, this assertion is accurate, and health care providers and educators can be properly proud of this achievement.

Despite this history of success, or perhaps because of it, increasing numbers of voices are expressing concern about the potential for falling standards of care.[29] Three main areas of concern stand out. In America's largest cities, many hospitals, doctors, visiting nurses associations, and other parts of the delivery system are overwhelmed by the amount of need they face.[30] Many providers have simply abandoned these communities, thereby increasing the pressures on those who remain. Inner city communities have very high percentages of racial and ethnic minorities, populations that are also statistically underinsured and at higher risk for health care problems. This problem, typified by the day-to-day crisis atmosphere of many hospitals in New York City, Chicago, and Los Angeles, are continuous with the larger problem of failing educational and social services in inner cities in the United States. Providers in these communities face situations of triage on a regular basis, situations that can only be compared with those encountered in warfare. Even with the best equipment, it is hard to see how such overstressed institutions and professionals can maintain standards of care comparable to those routinely met in America's suburban hospitals.

Second, pressures to contain costs are forcing cutbacks and downsizing throughout the health care sector.[31] The average length of stay in a hospital has become dangerously short, and the number of nurses per hospital bed has been sharply reduced. How long both phenomena can continue without creating quality problems is an open question. In addition, oversight by third-party payers has become far more aggressive. Many doctors who fought insurers for exceptions for their patients in the mid-1980s have capitulated to the constant pressures by payers and administrators. In many hospitals an uncomplicated delivery now "requires" only twenty-four hours of inpatient admission, an amount of time that would have been considered dangerously short just a few years ago. The general movement of the site of care away from the hospital and into the home and other less intensive community locations is itself cause for concern. The hospital is a very public institution, with highly developed mechanisms for ensuring quality. With the explosion of home health care, surgicenters, and free-standing diagnostic centers, it is unclear whether hospital systems for maintaining quality can be replicated for these more private, decentralized locations. If they cannot be, then quality may suffer and the decline may be very hard to document.

Finally, there are disturbing signs that many health care professionals, especially doctors, are experiencing significant occupational burnout.[32] Large percentages of contemporary doctors would not choose to enter the profession again knowing what they know at this point in their careers, nor would they recommend the profession to a child or relative.[33] Such sentiments represent a dangerous degree of disaffection. It is hard to see how individuals with this sort of alienation can continue to maintain appropriately high standards of quality. Many factors may account for this demoralization: increased cost-containment pressures, more regulation from payers and government, a general loss of independence of practice, lowered public prestige, downward pressure on salaries, and increased legal hazards in the working environment. Few of these factors are likely to change in a more positive direction in the near future. Indeed, many are sure to worsen. Therefore, vigilance must continue by both the profession and the general public in monitoring the relationship between doctors' attitudes and their quality of care. Professional satisfaction may be subjective and intangible, but it is an important, perhaps a central, ingredient in sustaining the ability to care properly both for patients and for oneself.

This litany of challenges facing the American health care system would be daunting enough were problems of access, cost, and quality three independent areas that could be addressed on their own terms; but this is plainly not the case. These three areas interact in a more or less direct fashion. Frequently, the consequence of addressing a problem under one heading is to worsen problems under another heading. Some obvious methods of enhancing access, for example, can only come about with either increased costs or diminished quality. Generally speaking, one cannot serve more people except by paying more or by being willing to accept lower standards. The obvious strategies for containing costs are to serve fewer people or to provide them with fewer and lower quality services. Similarly, maintaining or increasing high standards of quality means increasing costs unless fewer people are served. Thus the goals of universal access, cost containment, and quality enhancement appear to be linked in a zero-sum relationship. Making an advance on one goal seems to threaten progress in one or both of the other goals. Yet neither universal access, serious cost containment, nor the maintenance of high quality standards can be easily dismissed as a genuine goal because each represents its own moral imperative.

In practical terms, reflection on this intellectual difficulty could be paralyzing. Simply put, it could lead to the conclusion that health care reform is an impossible task. The intellectual and practical challenge here is real and must be borne in mind as efforts are made to return to the health care reform agenda. Nevertheless, these challenges do not make true health care reform a logically impossible task or the equivalent of a contradiction in terms. In fact, the problem appears in an entirely different light when the relative successes of other nations' health care systems are noted. No nation has a perfect health care system, and each has to grapple in its own way with the same access–cost–quality triad. Nonetheless, the striking fact is that every comparable industrial democracy in the world covers all its citizens, spends less than the United States to do so, and has achieved a level of quality generally acceptable to their own public.[34] The examples of these other countries—nations as diverse as Italy, Canada, and Japan—constitute evidence that the road to health care reform, though difficult, is not impossible to travel.

Plainly, success for the United States cannot come from simply copying the efforts of other nations, although much can be learned from them. Instead, the United States must return to health care reform on terms consistent with American experiences and traditions. Chief among these are the moral values Americans should and do use in the health care arena, the values that define in the most fundamental way what health care should be and what can reasonably be expected from it. Progress toward the goals of universal access, meaningful cost containment, and high standards of care must occur within an explicit acknowledgment of the links between these goals and Americans' most important moral values.

Notes

1. Jane H. White, "Health System Changes in the Absence of National Reform," *Health Progress* 57, no. 10 (1994): 10–12, 16.
2. Charles J. Dougherty, "Ethical Values at Stake in Health Care Reform," *JAMA*, 268, no. 17 (1992): 2409–12; Reinhard Priester, "A Values Framework for Health System Reform," *Health Affairs* 11, no. 1 (1992): 84–107.

3. Robert J. Blendon et al., "The American Public and the Critical Choices for Health Care Reform," *JAMA* 271, no. 19 (1994): 1539-44. Polls show that the public gives its highest support to sin taxes on alcohol, cigarettes, guns, and ammunition as a means to fund universal coverage, taxes least likely to raise the revenue required.

4. Erick Eckholm, "While Congress Remains Silent, Health Care Transforms Itself," *New York Times*, 18 December 1994, pp. 1, 22; and Katherine Swartz, *The Medically Uninsured* (Washington, D.C.: The Urban Institute, 1989).

5. Robert Blendon, Mollyann Brodie, and John Benson, "What Should Be Done Now That National Health System Reform is Dead?" *JAMA* 273, no. 3 (1995): 243-44.

6. Katherine Swartz, "Dynamics of People Without Health Insurance," *JAMA* 271, no. 1 (1994): 64-66.

7. P. Cotton, "Preexisting Conditions 'Hold Americans Hostage' to Employers and Insurance," *JAMA* 265, no. 19 (1991): 2451-53.

8. Alvin L. Schnorr, "Job Turnover—A Problem with Employer-Based Health Care," *The New England Journal of Medicine* 323, no. 8 (1990): 543-45.

9. Danielle A. Dolenc and Charles J. Dougherty, "DRGs: The Counterrevolution in Financing Health Care," *Hastings Center Report* 15, no. 3 (1985): 19-29.

10. See, e.g., "Peter Franks, Carolyn M. Clancy, and Martha R. Gold, "Health Insurance and Mortality," *JAMA* 270, no. 6 (1993): 737-41; Jack Hadley, Earl Steinberg, and Judith Feder, "Comparison of Uninsured and Privately Insured Hospital Patients, *JAMA* 265, no. 3 (1991): 374-79.

11. See, e.g., K. Shaw, S. Selbst, and F. Gill, "Indigent Children Who Are Denied Care in the Emergency Department," *Annals of Emergency Medicine* 19, no. 1 (1990): 59-62; and E. Olsen "No Room at the Inn: A Snapshot of an American Emergency Room," *Stanford Law Review* 46, no. 2 (1994): 449-501.

12. Robert Blendon, Mollyann Brodie, and John Benson, *JAMA* (1995): 243.

13. Stephen Long and M. Susan Marquis, "The Uninsured 'Access Gap' and the Cost of Universal Coverage," *Health Affairs* 13, no. 2, (1994): 211-20, esp. p. 215.

14. Robert Blendon et al. "Medicaid Beneficiaries and Health Reform," *Health Affairs* 12, no. 1 (1993): 132-43.

15. Peter Franks, Paul A. Nutting, and Carolyn Clancy, "Health Care Reform, Primary Care, and the Need for Research," *JAMA* 270, no. 12 (1993): 1449-53.

16. Charlene Harrington et al., "A National Long-term Care Program for the United States, *JAMA* 266, no. 21 (1991): 3023-29; for an international perspective, see United States General Accounting Office, *Long-Term Care: Other Countries Tighten Budgets While Seeking Better Access*," GAO/HEHS-94-154, August 1994.

17. Nancy S. Jenker and Robert A. Pearlman, "Medical Futility: Who Decides?" *Archives of Internal Medicine* 152 (June 1992): 1140-44.

18. Robert Blendon and Karen Donelan, "The Public and the Emerging Debate Over National Health Insurance," *The New England Journal of Medicine* 232, no. 3 (1990): 208-12.

19. Robert Blendon et al. "The Beliefs and Values Shaping Today's Health Reform Debate," *Health Affairs* 13, no. 1 (1994): 274-84.

20. James P. Hadley, "Overview," *Health Care Financing Review* 15, no. 1 (1993): 1-5.

21. Bob Kerrey and Philip Hofschire, "Hidden Problems in Current Health-Care Financing and Potential Changes," *American Psychologist* 48, no. 3 (1993): 261-64.

22. J. Barber, "Telling the Public the Real Health Cost Story," *Hospitals* 66, no. 12 (1990): 68.

23. Paul Weiler, Joseph Newhouse, and Howard Hiatt, "Proposal for Medical Liability Reform," *JAMA* 267, no. 17 (1992): 2355-58.

24. Steffie Woolhandler and David Himmelstein, "The Deteriorating Administrative Efficiency of the U.S. Health Care System," *The New England Journal of Medicine* 324, no. 18 (1991): 1253-57.

25. John K. Iglehart, "Medicare," *The New England Journal of Medicine* 327, no. 20 (1992): 1467-72; and Robin Toner, "Groups Rally to Fight Medicare Cuts," *New York Times* 18 December 1994, p. 19.

26. John K. Iglehart, "Medicaid," *The New England Journal of Medicine* 328, no. 12 (1993): 896-900.

27. See, e.g., S. Butler, "A Tax Reform Strategy to Deal with the Uninsured," *Journal of American Medical Association* 265, no. 19 (1991): 2541-44; and David Kendall and Will Marshall, "Health Reform, Meet Tax Reform," *The American Prospect* no. 21 (Spring 1995): 74-78.

28. Eli Ginzberg, *The Road to Reform* (New York: The Free Press, 1994): 21-39.

29. See, e.g., Eleanor Chelimsky, "The Political Debate About Health Care: Are We Losing Sight of Quality?" *Science* 262 (October 22, 1993): 525-28.

30. E.g., E. Friedman et al., "The Sagging Safety Net: Emergency Departments on the Brink of Crisis," *Hospitals* 66, no. 4 (1992): 26-40.

31. Eleanor Chelimsky, "The Political Debate About Health Care: Are We Losing Sight of Quality?" *Science* 262 (October 22, 1993): 525-28.

32. G. Deckard, M. Meterko, and D. Field, "Physician Burnout: An Examination of Personal, Professional, and Organizational Relationships," *Medical Care* 32, no. 7 (1994): 745-54.

33. One poll found that fourteen percent of one thousand doctors interviewed would definitely not enter the profession knowing what they now know about the practice of medicine; another twenty-five percent probably would not. Lawrence Altman and Elisabeth Rosenthal, "Changes in Medicine Bring Pain to Healing Profession," *New York Times*, 18 February 1990, pp. 1 and 20.

34. William Glaser, "The United States Needs a Health System Like Other Counties," *JAMA* 270, no. 8 (1993): 980-84.

2

Values

Foundations

Because this is a book about the values that do and should shape American health care, it will be useful at the outset to clarify insofar as possible the nature and function of values. In its broadest expression, a value is a desired state of affairs, a situation or condition of worth.[1] Some values are instrumental.[2] Their role lies chiefly in service to another value or set of values. Efficiency in a hospital, for example, is typically valued because it contributes to the value or values that direct the organization itself by facilitating the provision of its services. The value of revenue in the hospital budget is generally instrumental in the sense that the primary good of money is its usefulness in funding hospital services. There are numerous examples of instrumental values. They can generally be identified as excellences in processes or media of exchange. Thus, hospitality can be an instrumental value, as can clarity in organizational communication.

The more primitive kind of value refers to states of affairs that are experienced as intrinsically worthy. The value of physical health, natural beauty, or works of art is inherent in experiencing them. Significant human relationships of caring or healing are values that are prized for themselves. Experiences of pleasure, happiness, and a sense of satisfaction are all *intrinsic* values.

Although often helpful, this distinction between intrinsic and instrumental values is neither sharp nor definitive. Efficiency, for example, which is generally instrumental, can also be valued in itself. One might, for instance, find the overall goals of an outpatient sports clinic to be of little or no value and yet regard the efficiency of the clinic as estimable. Money can also become an intrinsic value, as is clearly the case for collectors of rare coins but is also evident in the generally perverse yet real values of the miser who hoards money for its own sake or the CEO driven to maximize margin.

The distinction between intrinsic and instrumental can be eroded in the opposite direction as well. Values that are typically intrinsic can sometimes play instrumental roles. Experiences of beauty can be useful in the service of other values, for example, in pastoral care, enhancing cleanliness, or creating an image of credibility and respect. In addition to being valued in themselves, relationships of care and healing can be instrumentally related to other values, such as building healthy families and communities and fostering professional careers. Because they are the desiderata in both end states and processes, values display all the variety of the changing and interpenetrating goals and processes of life itself.

The operation of values, in the most basic sense of activity drawn toward desired goals or processes, is evident throughout nature. In this sense, all living things seem to value life and maintaining a certain harmony with their environment. Animal behavior seems to display a characteristic set of values that includes survival, reproduction, and a preference for the company of members of the same species. Higher animals display a more complex network of values, including (in some cases) curiosity, playfulness, and loyalty to mates, offspring, and clan. Values pervade human existence. From the profound to the trivial, much of human life is structured around the pursuit of activities or states taken to be desirable in themselves or desirable as means.

Regarded naturally, values provide direction in life, driving humans toward goals and away from threats. No doubt they provide motives for behaviors that are linked to our survival as a species. Culturally, values provide standards for measuring success or failure, progress or decline. They are the content of our public symbols for the best and the worst in our social life. Existentially, values are a source of meaning in life. They provide individuals and groups with a sense of purpose that goes beyond the struggles or delights of the here and now. Values link the smallness, temporality, and incompleteness of all things human to grandeur, to permanence, and to the ideal.

Moral Values

The values most important in assessing the health care system are moral values, which are typically thought to be more significant than other values, to be controlling or overriding of other values. People with strong moral values commonly abstain from enjoying other valued conditions when those conditions or the steps necessary to attain them are thought to be incompatible with their own moral values. A morally committed doctor, for example, will refrain from recommending an unnecessary treatment even when to do so would be profitable. Moral values typically have a connection to the welfare of people or groups of people, to human relationships, or to aspects of personality; thus, kindness to children, fidelity to patients, and professional integrity are moral values.

Identification of moral values is facilitated by the presence of certain characteristic concepts and vocabulary. Moral values are generally at stake when states of affairs or relationships or conditions of a personality are described as good, bad, better, or worse. Moral values are also generally at stake when actions are described as "wrong" in the sense of being prohibited, "right" in the sense of being obligatory (do the right thing) or in the sense of permissible (the act was right). "Ought" and its cognates "must," and "should" are also markers of moral values. For contemporary Americans, the language of rights (she had a right to it; his rights were violated) is also generally an indication of the presence of moral values.

Again, it is important to note that this distinction between moral and nonmoral values, although helpful, is not definitive conceptually or always clear in specific contexts. Kindness to one's children, for example, can be both a moral value and a personal preference. A doctor's fidelity to patients can express a moral value or simply a prudent business strategy. Likewise, professional integrity can be a moral value and also the best way to avoid accusations of medical malpractice. Moreover, words that sometimes mark moral values can also have other nonmoral uses. A judgment that an evening was "a good time" or a "bad experience" may or may not involve moral values. Words like right, wrong, and should can also express arbitrary social conventions with little moral content (the fork should be to the left of the plate). Some assertions of rights may also have little connection to moral value, being only linguistic moves in an adversarial social relationship. "Rights" can also be used in a narrowly political sense in which moral content can be minimal or absent.

The situation is made more complex by the fact that moral values can also shade into values that are more properly regarded as legal, religious, or personal. The law embodies a great deal of moral value in both its substantive positions and its processes.[3] Nonetheless, it is frequently important to distinguish what is primarily a matter of moral value from what is primarily a matter of legal value. As a general rule, legal values are typically set within an authoritative, written context. Acts of legislation, court decisions, civil and penal procedures all embody important legal values that can be distinguished from moral values. Religious values also have considerable overlap with moral values for many people, perhaps for most.[4] Helpful distinguishing marks of the specifically religious include explicit reference to God or interpretations of God's will, sacred writings, rituals, and other religious traditions. Moral values also can shade into personal value. The two realms are often difficult to distinguish in practical contexts. One frequently helpful difference is between the universalizing tendency of moral values and the idiosyncratic character of the personal.[5] A personal value might be expressed as, "I want a job with comprehensive health insurance," whereas a related moral value might assert, "All jobs should provide comprehensive health insurance."

Features of Moral Values

Although admittedly making sharp identification of moral values is difficult, some typical features of these values are still worth noting. In addition to their focus on desired states of human welfare, relationships, and personality, moral values typically share seven features: ubiquity, vagueness, implicitness, spontaneity, emotional charge, practicality, and depth.

Moral values are ubiquitous. This feature can easily be overlooked because moral dilemmas or controversies appear to punctuate everyday experience only rarely. Controversies about the disposition of frozen embryos, for example, or the justice of cuts in Medicaid turn on moral values and arise only periodically. Whereas such large-scale issues plainly involve moral values, they ought not blind us to the moral values that permeate ordinary experience. Value preferences about states of affairs, human relationships, and personality shape our daily judgments and actions. For example, choices about lifestyle or concerning the amount of time allotted to competing activities involve moral values because they represent a prioritization of better and worse. Individuals inspecting their habits and lifestyle for health implications are faced with significant everyday moral choices. A nurse deciding how much time to spend with each inpatient or with each family during home visits makes numerous moral choices. Countless daily actions are shaped by the sense of who a person wants to be and by the importance attached to relationships with others. Once the moral values in these everyday realities are noticed, their presence can be seen virtually everywhere.

Some moral values are quite specific and concrete. It may be very important in itself, for example, to comfort a child in pain. More often, moral values are vague. What is the precise content, for example, to be associated with the much-discussed issue of "family values"? Some Americans may have a relatively clear set of ideals that fall under this description: raising children in families with two married parents, traditional roles for wife and mother, religious practice and education, self-reliance, and other ideals. Even in this relatively clear agenda, however, room exists for an endless variety of interpretations. Do family values cover extended families and step-parents, mothers taking on new roles as home teachers, non-Western religions? How much self-reliance is demanded by this notion of family values? Should Medicare and Medicaid be rejected, for example, or modern health care itself, given all its public support?

Outside this politically charged conception of family values is even greater vagueness. Many Americans identify with the term family values in the sense that it summarizes substantial commitments in their lives; yet they do not interpret it to mean some or all of the above. Nontraditional families can develop the same emotional bonding and sense of responsibility for one another as do the more traditional family units. Many working women, some in quite nontraditional roles, combine careers with deep commitments to their families. Many contemporaries have allegiances to new religions or to new interpretations of traditional religions. Finally, active support from others, including government, may be the only means of survival for many families, thereby limiting the role of self-reliance in this understanding of family values. Medicare, Medicaid, and various supports from health care and social work professionals are lifelines for many families. Therefore, even in the context of this noteworthy and much-discussed example of values, there is considerable room for many interpretations and applications.

It is important to add that vagueness in moral values is not in itself a flaw, the way vagueness typically would be in law, mathematics, or commercial transactions. The aspirational dimension of values makes them properly indistinct because it links judgment and action to ideal states that can be only partially and imaginatively understood and felt. Therefore, this vagueness in meaning, though sometime frustrating, is often an important positive dimension of moral values, allowing and even promoting multiple articulations of the ideal at hand and thereby offering different directions from which the ideal can be approximated.

Moral values are also generally more implicit than explicit. Sometimes controversy or the need for clarity in a specific context can make a moral value explicit. A person can become quite conscious of a motivation with respect to a desired state of affairs or process; but this consciousness is more the exception than the rule. Many people's most important moral values are seldom, if ever, made explicit to others or to themselves. People live with or through their values, rarely thinking explicitly about them. The medical records clerk who stays after hours to finish an important project many never have an explicit thought about loyalty to co-workers. Nonetheless, this moral value is implicit in such behavior. This feature of values, along with the inherent vagueness already identified, can make the process of clarifying or articulating values difficult. If the clerk in question never has the explicit motivation of being loyal to co-workers, the dominant value shaping this clerk's action may in fact be something else. It could be an unspoken understanding that some after-hours work is part of the job or a sense of pride in seeing a project through to the end. Indeed, these and other factors may coexist with the implicit moral value of loyalty to co-workers.

Moral values are also spontaneous. They typically arise and shape behavior without needing to be forced. In the vast majority of applications, action with respect to a moral value has a certain intuitive obviousness and naturalness. Commitment to family values or to caring for the needs of children, for example, may be the moral values that best describe the behavior of a parent who leaves work to attend to a sick child; but leaving work probably seems the obviously right thing to do for the parent, even if no notion of right versus wrong, no conscious thought of moral values ever arises or enters the situation.

Again, high-profile moral debates can obscure this point. Sometimes a moral value must be forced onto a situation because competing values seem to apply and a choice must be made. Perhaps no precedent exists for the application of any value to a new situation. Should frozen embryos be considered persons or property, for example? Sometimes choice concerning moral values follows a moment of difficult internal or public debate, but these are the rare occasions, the exceptions. The operation of most moral values are like the spontaneous movements of a healthy person. By contrast, the rare but remarkable cases of tortured choice or a lengthy public debate are like the movement of someone with an impaired limb. In the former case, there is spontaneity; in the latter, there must be deliberate, often painful effort.

Moral values are emotionally charged, many having obvious affective roots. The construction of emotions related to morality is evident in early childhood development. Adults convey important moral values to children through stories with moral pathos, like "the boy who cried wolf." Adults also shape childhood behaviors through systematic rewards and punishments, including praising and blaming. These efforts guarantee that important moral values enter a child's consciousness linked with strong feelings. From a parent's point of view, an indispensable part of moral education is leading a child to feel good about being good and to feel bad about being bad. Early formative experiences are followed in youth by stories of heros and saints, the approval or disapproval of authorities, and the emotion-laden judgments of peers in conversation and gossip. The emotional link with moral values continues throughout adult life in the arts and entertainment, in the socialization of careers, and in the general interpenetration of thinking and feeling in the lives of individuals and communities. The emotional dimension is important to bear in mind in any explicit discussion of moral values. Criticism of another's moral values can be deeply offensive because of the many emotional associations involved. This helps to explain why arguments about moral values can be so divisive. The debate on abortion, for example, involves not only differing cognitive views about the procedure itself, but also a clash of deeply divergent feelings about life and choice.

Moral values are also practical. They guide actions, shape habits, and give direction to the lives of individuals and whole societies. Genuine commitment to a preferred state of affairs typically entails the choice of actions that more closely realize the ideal when such actions are possible. Values move people by attraction. The inherent admirability of a moral value draws choices and actions toward itself, other things being equal. Of course, moral values can be "held" hypocritically so that no real action toward them is intended or so that actions taken are inimical to the values allegedly held. A leader in the small business community, for example, may publicly espouse the moral importance of providing health care for all Americans and yet work assiduously against every practical means of attaining that goal. Even in cases of hypocrisy, however, moral values are not practically ineffective. Hypocrites' real moral values are displayed through their actions. The problem of hypocrisy lies not in the ineffectiveness of moral values, but in the incompatibility of values espoused verbally and those evident in practice. The practical dimensions of moral values also raise the stakes in cases of moral disagreement, because one who holds a value does not simply want that value recognized intellectually, but wants the value realized in practice.

Finally, moral values are deep. Compared with other kinds of values, except for some religious and personal values, moral values tend to be more profoundly important to both people and societies. They provide some of the richest sources of meaning by orienting imperfect beings to ideals. The moral value of integrity, for example, can be a deeply important commitment because a person with that value not only wants to be, but in imagination already is, a person of complete integrity. One's sense of self and degree of self-esteem is shaped by these ideal conceptions of what the self wants to be and how close an approximation the real self is to its ideal. In one sense a person just *is* that individual's most important and firmly held values.

Because of this depth, moral values are often closely linked to religious values in providing a sense of profundity and purpose in life. Depth also distinguishes moral values from most personal values, which can be self-consciously capricious. Like religious values, moral values intend a kind a objectivity typically missing in personal values. In monotheistic religions, for example, God is not just a god but *the* God. By contrast, a career is a personal value. It is not *the* career. In this respect, important moral values operate more like religious values than like personal values. Moral values have a depth that expresses this note of objectivity. Those who hold professional integrity to be an important moral value, for example, typically regard it as a fundamental insight into professional relationships. Integrity is not a way to behave; it is *the* way.

Origins and Influences

It will be helpful to explore further the origins of moral value.[6] The context of early childhood education has already been touched on. Parents frequently educate children explicitly on moral values by praising kindness and condemning cruelty, building healthy habits, and providing a raft of morally charged explanations, rules, and stories. Perhaps even more important are the indirect, unconscious moral values that are "taught" through the parent's own behavior and the structure of the family environment. Siblings, teachers, and friends play similar roles.

The general culture is also an important source of moral values for each of us. Substantive and pervasive moral values are taught explicitly by all of society's major institutions, most especially by the law and the general patterns of life and behavior. Contemporary mass media, a powerful moral educator, sometimes teaches explicitly but nearly always willy nilly, as evidenced by the values implied and frequently taught explicitly in television talk shows, dramas, and situation comedies.

The important and pervasive moral instructions of culture are frequently disguised and become clear only when foreign or competing moral values come into view. The values most Americans now share about the emancipation of women, for example, go largely unnoticed despite their relatively recent vintage; but a film account of moral values on this topic in the last century or a visit to a nation where fundamentalist Islamic traditions dominate will throw American value commitments into sharp relief. Similarly, one can easily forget how much contemporary American culture teaches about racial fairness until an encounter with a novel about antebellum slavery, a film about nineteenth century Indian Wars, or a documentary on the internment of Japanese-American citizens during World War II.

The strong connections between moral values and religious values have already been noted. Considerable overlap continues between the general moral values of secular life in America and the moral values that derive more or less directly from the dominant Judeo-Christian tradition.[7] Of course, this is no coincidence. The contemporary secular world evolved from the more explicitly religious society over generations of European and American experience. Many Americans maintain a strong link with that religious tradition. For many, secular moral values are a lingua franca needed for communicating in a society with increasing religious diversity. Their own personal encounter with the moral values important to American secular culture is grounded in an explicitly religious context that provides a different and, for them, a fuller framework for appreciating these values. It is also true that the moral values at the heart of secular life in the United States have affected and shaped religious institutions and values as well. American notions of fairness and equality that evolved in secular struggles and in the law have become commonplace expectations in many religious communities, even those with long traditions of different value commitments.

It is also important to note the rising significance on the American scene of religions outside the Judeo–Christian tradition: Islam, Buddhism, Native American spirituality, and others.[8] Many Americans identify with no religious traditions at all, and some consciously reject all religion. Nevertheless, the moral values of the nation through the end of the twentieth century have been shaped more by the Judeo–Christian religious tradition than by any other. Also dominating, as a matter of fact, are political and cultural movements drawn from European sources, especially the European Enlightenment of the seventeenth and eighteenth centuries.[9] These are our common cultural roots. The growing numbers of Americans with non-European ancestry certainly have introduced other influences and will continue to do. The fact remains, nonetheless, that important influences on national moral values, especially those related to health care, are the Judeo–Christian religious tradition and the European Enlightenment. These observations are not meant to diminish or disparage in any way the important contributions of other religious and sociopolitical traditions to the formation of contemporary American moral values, but only to assert the obvious historical facts and thereby make that history available for reflection and analysis.

Conflicts Between Values

Acknowledgment of diverse streams of moral values in American life opens the question of conflicts between values. Even if all Americans had the same moral and religious values, opportunities would still arise for differing interpretations of fundamental values and differing applications to changing circumstances. Religious leaders from the same faiths frequently disagree among themselves. Family members raised in the same household can have differing sets of values, sometimes profoundly so. Add to this general fact about the vagueness of shared values the increasing diversity in the United States, and there is endless possibility for dispute on fundamental moral values. Many of the most important values, for example, of a contemporary American feminist with New Age religious affiliations will be in direct opposition to those of a fundamentalist Christian or Orthodox Jew.

Even where there is considerable consensus on core moral values, challenges are created by dissenters. The vast majority of Americans would find the values of a member of the Ku Klux Klan perverse, but that person is still motivated by moral values. Even if such values are inconsistent with those of the majority, they are still moral in the sense of a deep normative commitment to a preferred state of affairs–to the way that person believes things ought to be. This fact reveals two meanings of the term moral values. The usual meaning, which suggests a normative consensus, is that moral values are those affirmed by my group; and the other meaning, which is descriptive, is that moral values are those taken to be moral by any person or group. In this second, descriptive sense, Nazis, drug gangs, and international terrorists have moral values, even if their moral values happen to be repugnant to those of most Americans. From this particular normative perspective, Nazi values are immoral, but they are nonetheless moral values in function. By understanding moral values in this descriptive way, there can be vast and unbridgeable gulfs between peoples' moral values and on issues that truly make a difference in private and public lives.

Faced with the awesome potential for conflict of moral values, what strategies exist for reconciliation or working out a *modus vivendi*? One obvious strategy, and one that has been important in shaping American history, is a commitment to wide toleration of differences in moral values.[10] Thus, toleration operates as a second-level metavalue for accommodating a wide variety of substantive value differences. Associated with tolerance are a nest of other values, including civility, fair play, and the presumption of goodwill that operate to give toleration some practical bearing, especially in disputes about public policy.

Clearly, there must be limits to toleration. The need for police and for armies indicates that even in societies with traditions of a wide range of toleration, some behaviors are simply beyond toleration. As a general rule, the boundaries of a reasonable extension of toleration can be marked by values that undermine toleration itself. In a relatively free and diverse society, it is intolerance that is intolerable. Direct acts of violence against the innocent or advocacy of such acts are intolerant and therefore beyond the bounds of toleration. So, too, are other less aggressive, but still harmful, acts of intolerance, like racism and sexism; but the general insight that one need not, and should not, tolerate the intolerant can be hard to apply in practice. For example, is racially provocative speech best tolerated as a form of speech or best made illegal as an intolerable form of racism?

Other difficult ethical issues that turn on fundamental moral values can also escape the strategy of toleration. The abortion issue, for example, has become so difficult and so divisive because both sides view the other's position as beyond the normal bounds of toleration. One side sees the other as attempting to impose a religiously inspired interpretation of the beginning of life, whereas the other side sees the first as endorsing direct violence against innocent life. Interpretations of toleration alone will not resolve disputes of this fundamental character. Nonetheless, as a general rule, it remains helpful to mark the boundaries of toleration at intolerant behavior.

Moral Relativism

There is an important implication of America's increasing diversity that deserves careful attention. The growing presence of Americans with differing moral values raises the difficult issues of moral relativism. Are there any universal truths in morality, bottom lines of behavior that everyone should share? Or is every moral value relative to a culture or an individual? A descriptive form of relativism is obviously true: There is a plurality of moral values in the United States, although there may be much more agreement on fundamentals than is allowed by some descriptive relativists.

Moral relativism goes beyond acknowledgment of the fact of a plurality of moral values, however.[11] It makes the normative claim that, given the diversity of views, all moral values are relative to a time, a place, a person, a context. If this is so, then no one *should* assert the validity of their moral values beyond their own cultural circumstances or even beyond the immediacy of their own personal circumstances. In essence, this is the view that moral values can have no objectivity, no truth beyond the relative conditions that give rise to them. Ironically, this position often amounts in practice to a dogmatic relativism, that is to say, a relativism about all moral positions *except* moral relativism itself, which is held as an absolute. Dogmatic normative relativism asserts that no person, regardless of circumstances, should claim more for that person's individual moral values than validity in a given time and place for a particular group or for a specific person. The irony is especially obvious when put this way: It is always wrong to judge anyone else's moral values or choices to be wrong.

This view cannot be accepted in this extreme form for at least three reasons. First, it is obviously inconsistent with itself. One cannot consistently claim to know objectively for all time that there are no objective, for-all-time truths. If all moral views are relative, then so is moral relativism, which means that the claim that all moral views are relative to a time and a place is a judgment that is itself relative to a time and place. The proper response, therefore, to the relativist who claims that moral judgments are true only for the person who makes them is the rejoinder that this view is true only for the relativist.

Second, there is a small, perhaps a vanishingly small, step from this agnosticism about values to outright value atheism: moral nihilism. The nihilist holds that nothing is really of value, that there is no validity to any claim about some conditions being better or worse than others; but nihilism, if genuinely believed, strips away all the meaning that moral values give to life. If nothing is better than anything else, then life is equivalent to death, healing neither better nor worse than harming, and a war on cancer morally indistinguishable from a war on foreigners or immigrants. In such a world, a human being is, to use Jean-Paul Sartre's trenchant phrase "a useless passion." It literally "makes no difference whether one becomes a leader of nations or gets drunk alone."[12]

Finally, there is a fundamental practical problem with this extreme form of moral relativism. It entails that there cannot be any moral validity to some uses of force. The notion of legitimate authority is lost and all force becomes sheer power.[13] The police officer with a gun is the moral equivalent of the gang member with a gun; opening a chest cavity with a scalpel for heart surgery is no different from opening a chest cavity with a switchblade in a robbery. Even legal prohibitions against murder, rape, and the abuse of research subjects amount to little more than an arbitrary imposition of preference, the ability of the powerful to force their will on others. Could any society survive if large numbers of its members held this view? How in such a society would any constraints on violence be possible, except those born in violence themselves? Under such circumstances life might resemble Thomas Hobbes' characterization of society before organized political authority: "solitary, poor, nasty, brutish, and short."[14]

The challenge implied here is to craft an understanding of value pluralism that does not amount to an extreme form of relativism, one that recognizes the legitimacy of moral diversity without dissolving the bases for all moral meaning and standards; this can be done.[15] Pluralism is the acknowledgment that a human life can be lived well on the bases of many differing values and many differing orderings of overlapping sets of values; but pluralism loses its significance without the implied objectivity of the standard of a human life well lived, of the overarching sense of human thriving toward which values aim. It is this objective norm, however difficult to determine in particular circumstances, that provides the justification for the metavalue of toleration, the grounds for rejecting the nihilism of extreme relativism, and the basis for hope that moral progress is possible.

Individualism

There is a less extreme form of relativism that is easier to recognize because it is widely influential in contemporary American life, a relativism that attempts to avoid the acrimonies of public discussion about moral values by adopting an insular form of individualism.[16] It holds that all or most key choices about moral values should be left to individuals. Insular individualism is less theoretically pretentious than dogmatic moral relativism; it does not claim that there is no moral truth, but it is more influential in practice. Its general attitude is captured in such easygoing slogans as: "I do my thing. You do yours. As long no one gets hurt, everything is fine."

As attractive as this posture is to many Americans, it cannot be the whole truth about moral values. Many moral values have a clear social and public component that cannot be waived in favor of individualism. Whether Medicaid coverage should include bone marrow transplantation is hardly a matter that can be left to individuals. Moreover, individualism too often confuses the procedural question of who has the right to choose (the answer here frequently is the individual) with the substantive question of what is the right choice. Only an extreme relativist can hold that the individual who has the right to choose always makes the right choice—and only because the relativist believes that any choice becomes the right choice just because an individual has made it, in essence, that there really is no right choice.

In some cases, it clearly is the individual's choice to make because this person is most intimately affected, a choice by a competent adult about elective surgery, for example. Even in this kind of case, however, insular individualism frequently ignores two important moral features that surround and shape the context of choice. The first feature is the seeking and giving of advice. Suppose a patient facing a choice about surgery asks a friend for advice. "Do you think I should have the surgery?" The friend replies, "The choice is yours to make." This reply is accurate as far as it goes, but it is also unresponsive, even churlish. Replies of this sort reinforce the distance between individuals and undermine relationships of friendship and love. Giving and getting advice may often be troubling but are some of the activities that bind people together in moral communities, create shared standards, and build intimate relationships. What the patient requests is not a reminder about who has the right to choose; he or she presumably knows this. The request is for the other's advice about which choice is right.

The second feature often overlooked, or intentionally ignored, by insular individualists follows decisions. After any serious choice, evaluations and criticisms inevitably follow. Sometimes this is self-criticism. In important choices there are nearly always evaluations and criticisms by others: loved ones, friends, co-workers, fellow citizens, and others. Of course, such criticisms can be acrimonious and painful. Nevertheless, they play an important and indispensable role in morality and express an attitude of taking moral values seriously enough to be concerned when they are disregarded or misapplied. Neither the giving of advice nor subsequent criticism is possible conceptually when an insular individualism prevails, when "the choice is yours to make" exhausts the moral dimensions of choice. This form of individualism breaks the bonds of community and undermines the relationships and institutions that make the maintenance and transmission of moral values possible.

There is an important truth about relativism, however, that cannot be lost in these criticisms. Even though one can, and often must, act on moral values with conviction, it is not possible to know positively that one's values and these particular applications of them are the right ones. They can be believed to be right—often must be believed to be right—but they cannot be *known* to be so securely. Both personal and national histories testify to the fact that values that seemed so clear and compelling in the context of choice are often seen in retrospect as wrong, misapplied, or self-deceptive.[17] Therefore, a certain amount of modesty about moral values is appropriate. Humans are fallible, perhaps more so in ethics than elsewhere. Modesty in both content and tone must be combined, however, with a robust sense of the importance of moral values. There must be a willingness to critique the moral values in American life generally, especially those in an area as morally sensitive as health care. Diversity of views must be respected, goodwill cultivated, and the real possibility of error admitted. At the same time, though, the values that have and do dominate American health care must be analyzed, criticized, and the best among them pruned, preserved, and promoted.

Notes

1. See, e.g., R. Attfield, *A Theory of Value and Obligation* (London: Croom Held Ltd, 1987).
2. Dougherty, "Ethical Values at Stake in Health Care Reform," pp. 2409–12.
3. H. L. A. Hart, *Law, Liberty, and Morality* (Stanford, California: Stanford University Press, 1963).
4. See, generally, J. Roland Pennock and John W. Chapman, eds., *Religion, Morality, and the Law* (New York: New York University Press, 1988).
5. Tom Beauchamp and James Childress, *The Principles of Biomedical Ethics*, 4th ed. (New York: Oxford University Press, 1994), p. 26.
6. For a more extended framework, see David Carr, *Educating the Virtues: An Essay on the Philosophical Psychology of Moral Development and Education* (New York: Routledge, 1991).
7. Robert Bellah et al., *Habits of the Heart* (Berkeley, California: University of California Press, 1985), pp. 27–51; and Donald Joy, ed. *Moral Development*

Foundations: Judeo-Christian Alternatives to Piaget and Kohlberg (Nashville, Tennessee: Abingdon, 1983).

8. E. Allen Richardson, *Strangers in This Land: Pluralism and the Response to Diversity* (New York: Pilgrim Press, 1988).

9. Ernst Cassirer, *The Philosophy of the Enlightenment*, trans. by Fritz Koelln and James Pettegrove (Boston: Beacon Press, 1955); and Garry Wills, *Explaining America: The Federalist* (Garden City, N.Y.: Doubleday, 1981).

10. See, e.g., Robert Paul Wolff, Barrington Moore, and Herbert Marcuse, *A Critique of Pure Tolerance* (Boston: Beacon Press, 1965).

11. See, generally, Jack Meiland and Michael Krauz, eds., *Relativism, Cognitive and Moral* (Notre Dame, Ind.: University of Notre Dame Press, 1982).

12. Jean-Paul Sartre, *Being and Nothingness*, trans. Hazel Barnes (New York: Washington Square Press, 1966), pp. 784 and 797.

13. Jeffrey Reiman, *In Defense of Political Philosophy* (New York: Harper Torchbooks, 1972).

14. Thomas Hobbes, *Leviathan*, ed. by C. B. Macpherson (Baltimore: Penguin, 1976), p. 186.

15. See, for example, John Kekes, *The Morality of Pluralism* (Princeton, N.J.: Princeton University Press, 1993).

16. Charles J. Dougherty, "The Excesses of Individualism," *Health Progress* 73, no. 1 (January 1992): 22–28.

17. Mike Martin, *Self-Deception and Morality* (Lawrence, Kansas: University Press of Kansas, 1986).

3

Human Dignity

Foundations

One of the most important values at stake in the health care reform debate is human dignity.[1] This value provides a framework for appreciating the ethical commitment to respect individual persons; provides significance to the right to decline offered health care that is protected by informed consent; and is one basis for the demand for universal access to a basic package of health care benefits, for a right to health care. Human dignity is also the foundation for another value of significance to Americans: freedom.

In contemporary medical ethics, freedom, especially patient freedom, is often put forward as a rudimentary moral value or basic ethical principle under the heading of autonomy.[2] In this approach, respect for the self-determination of persons is a first premise of ethics, the practical expression of which is a right of noninterference by others. In medicine, this has come to mean a patient right of informed consent, especially the right to refuse unwanted treatments. These are important premises, but on this account they will be considered derivative in importance from a more fundamental moral premise: the value of the human person.

The reason for this prioritization is clear in many medical contexts in which there can be little or no meaningful applications of the notions of autonomy, self-determination, or freedom. Infants and young children, emergency patients under the influence of drugs or alcohol, persons with severe mental handicaps, and patients in shock or coma have no real autonomy; they cannot exercise reason and freedom. Other patients with serious mental and physical impairments, Alzheimer's and AIDS patients with dementia and persons with advanced Parkinson's and amyotrophic lateral sclerosis (ALS, or Lou Gehrig's disease), for example, have seriously diminished self-determination. If freedom is of paramount moral importance, their lives appear less worthy. If so, should their interests be taken seriously? They should be, it seems, only if the lives of such persons are considered valuable irrespective of the evident compromise in their freedom and other human capacities.

This insight suggests that before freedom can be valued, there is or should be a valuation of individual persons *as* persons. Presumption of this value would account for why so strong a moral demand is created by some of the least autonomous patients, including the chronically ill and dying. Any substantive moral value less than that applied to persons *as* persons would justify ignoring or even dispatching patients lacking the real expression of that value, whether it be freedom, productivity, self-awareness, being wanted by others, or whatever. Only a prior commitment to persons as persons regardless of their actual conditions makes sense of the traditional medical ethos and the natural moral sentiment to care for even the worst-off patients, to care especially for the worst-off patients. Furthermore, only a commitment to the value of persons as such allows for a robust sense of moral equality because any other substantive value not only eliminates some patients from the community of persons, but also allows, even encourages, a rank ordering of the value of persons. If, for example, self-determination is the most primitive moral value, then patients who are more self-determining are more valuable and those less self-determining are less valuable. If a sense of self is the key moral value, those with more of it are more worthy. If relations with others constitute the highest value, the poorer the human relations, the lesser the person. Only on the assumption that there is some universal value to persons that stands behind all other particular values can belief in the moral equality of humans be made meaningful. Only then can the multiple real differences among patients be dismissed as unimportant compared with the moral significance of each being a human person.

That superimposing value is human dignity. It is not, as the name often suggests, a belief in any special honor, power, or decorum that pertains to being human. All too clearly, this is not the case. In fact, the overwhelming empirical evidence is that the species and its individual members can be and often are dishonored and dishonorable, weak and vulnerable, graceless and indecent. Human dignity acts as a mask (*persona* is an actor's mask) that persons don to cover these frailties and failures with a moral assumption of profound individual worth. Dignity, then, is the value that humans have just by virtue of being human. In various traditions, commitment to human dignity is an existential choice, a conceptual discovery, or an act of faith. However arrived at, it functions as an assertion of the inner worth of all persons and therefore as the foundation for all other moral values and ethical principles pertaining to humans.

Roots

There are at least two roots to the American experience of human dignity or, more properly, the moral imperative to respect human dignity. The oldest, and in some respects the deepest root, is religious. The traditional Judeo–Christian belief in a personal and benevolent God with whom individuals have or can have a spiritual relationship gave rise historically to a special stress on the sanctity of each human life.[3] In this religious viewpoint, each person's life has a significance in a divine plan. Regardless of how clear or obscure that plan may appear to believers at any given time, belief in such an overarching meaningfulness provides a foundation for a special status for each person regardless of that person's station in life. It hardly needs to be added that this value never wholly controlled the behavior of nations or individual believers historically, nor does it now. Nevertheless, as a regulatory ideal, the value of human dignity provided important brakes on some of the worst human motivations and encouraged some of the more admirable. The value of human dignity in the Judeo–Christian religious tradition also served as a seed from which many significant liberation movements grew, including the American movements to abolish slavery in the nineteenth century and to establish a nonracial, uniform system of civil rights in the twentieth century.[4] In both cases, the use of religious language and insights centering on the inherent human dignity of each person made a powerful appeal to the American conscience.

The other root of the American experience of human dignity is the Enlightenment tradition.[5] The particular relevance of this tradition is its commitment to equality before the law, a system of equal human rights, and a wide range of individual freedom.[6] All these commitments are grounded in a conception of the civil inviolability of individuals. Many of the historically important persons who shaped the American expression of this European movement linked their commitment to the importance of each individual person to the Judeo–Christian tradition, or at least to a deistic interpretation of it. Thomas Jefferson, for example, summarized his political convictions this way: "I have sworn on the altar of God eternal hostility to every form of tyranny over the mind of man."[7] Despite religious origins, the Enlightenment tradition is most influential in the United States at the end of the twentieth century as a secular worldview. The religious view that human dignity derives from an act of divine creation outside the person is replaced by the view that human dignity is inherent in each human person. Individuals have dignity and human rights simply by virtue of being human.

Persons and Things

The secular Enlightenment account was given one of its best expressions by the German philosopher Immanuel Kant in the 1790s. Although he was a Christian Pietist, Kant's main contribution to understanding human dignity proceeded philosophically without direct appeal to religion. In Kant's view, to be a person is to be fundamentally different from a thing, the main difference lying in the realm of value.[8] The value of things is expressed in price. Two features of prices are especially important. First, prices are relative; some things are worth more than other things, some less. Relative price is affected by many factors, including usefulness, rarity, and demand. Because of these factors, the price or value of the very same thing can vary over time.

The other pertinent feature of price is that some, perhaps most, of the value of a thing is determined by realities outside the thing itself. Usefulness, for example, is external to a thing. A wheelchair derives much of its value, and therefore its price, by virtue of its function as a tool, in providing a conveyance for those who cannot walk. The economic laws of supply and demand also express the external character of the value of things. The same object, unchanged in any of its own properties, can become more or less valued, its price rising or falling, by virtue of changes in the economic environment. Aside from its usefulness, a wheelchair may become devalued if many wheelchairs like it are equally available. Similarly, its value may rise if wheelchairs are scarce and the need for them is great. So the value of things, as expressed in price, is both relative and external.

Kant held that the moral gulf between the value of persons and things lies in these two factors. Unlike things, the value of persons is neither relative nor external. Although persons can be valued differentially for their skills, experience, and other attributes, considered only as persons, their values cannot be compared or ranked. No number can be assigned to the value of one person compared with the value of the next. Because this is so, persons cannot be judged as having greater or less value. By Kant's account, the value of each person is incalculably great, absolute as opposed to relative. The meaning of this conviction becomes clearer when the second feature is considered. The value of persons is not external but internal. Therefore, considerations of usefulness or of the laws of supply and demand do not give rise to or shape the value of individual persons. Each person has an incalculably great and inherent value. For Kant, this was the essential meaning of human dignity: the absolute and intrinsic value of each person. Persons are literally priceless. They ought not to be treated as if they were merely things of relative and external value.

Rights

In political terms, the most significant expression of the American commitment to human dignity is the articulation and enforcement of a set of individual rights, beginning most prominently with the Bill of Rights.[9] From a contemporary perspective, American commitment to individual rights in the eighteenth and nineteenth centuries was deeply flawed by the exclusion of women and racial minorities from full membership in the political community. Despite this noteworthy failure, the Bill of Rights did help create a political culture that allowed for, perhaps made inevitable, the expansion of the political community to include all Americans. It also served as a model for similar developments worldwide. In fact, when historians provide a final assessment of the contribution of the United States to world civilization, legal enforcement of a comprehensive range of individual rights may well be regarded as the nation's most significant achievement.

It is important to note that the rights articulated in the eighteenth century in the Bill of Rights were largely negative rights, that is, rights to be free of interference by others, particularly by government.[10] Thus, the right of freedom of the press does not mean a right to publish a newspaper or even the right to secure a copy of one. The right of freedom of worship does not mean entitlement to a church or temple or a right to religious education. The right of freedom of assembly does not include a right of transportation to meet with others or a right to a place to meet. All these rights entail only a right to be free *from* interference with these activities if and when they can be undertaken on their own by individuals or groups. The government cannot prevent the publishing or reading of newspapers, religious worship or instruction, or assembly for any lawful purpose; but it need not foster any of these activities.

As a rule, negative rights are relatively well defined and inexpensive. They dictate what cannot be done. They can be respected by doing nothing, that is, by simply refraining from interfering with the lawful actions of others. Therefore, even though they can be demanding (people and governments *do* tend to interfere), negative rights are not costly in the literal sense. Government does not have to impose taxes or structure programs to ensure these rights; it just has to leave people alone.

Even in the eighteenth century, however, there was one area of exception to the generally negative character of American rights: the law. The U.S. Constitution guarantees a right to a speedy trial as well as a right to representation by a lawyer in cases of serious criminal charges.[11] These rights must be regarded as positive because they require considerable government action and funding. To respect these rights, government must build and maintain courthouses, employ judges, impanel juries, and secure the services of attorneys for persons accused of serious crimes.

Another positive right began to emerge in the early nineteenth century, based not on the U.S. Constitution, but on state constitutions and local customs: the right to education. From its beginnings in New England, the idea took hold through the century that children have a right to a basic education provided on a local basis with public support.[12] This positive right also required taxation and considerable action by state and local governments. Schools had to be built and maintained, teachers hired, texts and supplies secured, and so forth.

A general feature of positive rights is clear in this instance: Their scope is indistinct. Although there are inevitable boundary situations and conflicts about the scope of negative rights, they are relatively clear in application compared with the open-endedness of positive rights. The negative right, which forms the basis of the obligation to refrain from interfering with another's worship, creates a mandate that is fairly distinct: Do not interfere with another's religious practice. By contrast, a positive right to education raises innumerable theoretical and practical questions. How much education does a right to education entail? Is it simply a right to grade school, or does it include high school, college, professional education, and lifelong learning for adults? Who should pay for this right and how? How much direct involvement and control should government have? Who should determine the curriculum and standards for assessment? What about children with special needs? Do they have the same rights or more rights? Answers to these questions cannot be drawn directly from the concept of a right to education but must be answered by reference to evolving community needs, resources, and sensibilities.

Many European nations, especially those most influenced by the Judeo–Christian tradition and the Enlightenment, adopted a number of positive rights in the nineteenth and twentieth centuries,[13] including rights to education, housing, vocational training, employment or unemployment support, social services, and a right to health care or health insurance. Aside from rights to the legal system and to education, positive rights in the United States have been far more problematic. Because of a cultural disposition toward individualism and a general suspicion of government, Americans have been reluctant to guarantee positive rights.

Informed Consent

This American inclination to take the lead in negative rights and to be resistant on positive rights shows itself clearly in the health care arena. In effect, a positive right to some amount of health care is the prevailing norm in industrial democracies around the world. With the important exceptions of Medicare and Medicaid, the Veterans Administration, the Indian Health Service, and some other categorical programs, however, there is no positive right to health care in the United States. While Americans have resisted creation of a positive right to health care, at the same time they have been in the forefront in developing the essentially negative health care right of informed consent.[14]

Twentieth-century medicine in the United States abounds with revolutionary elements, especially in technology, pharmaceuticals, surgery, and innovative delivery systems; but there has been a cultural revolution in twentieth-century medicine that is rarely noted in spite of its profound character and effects. Consistent with the main tradition of Western medicine, U.S. medicine through the first half of the twentieth century was decidedly paternalistic. Because of doctors' knowledge, professional commitments, and social prestige, decision-making in health care generally meant following a doctor's orders or choosing to be noncompliant. Regardless of the patient's age, the doctor–patient relationship was much like that between a parent and child. The doctor/parent knew what was best for the patient/child and felt justified in imposing treatment decisions, withholding information, and even deceiving patients in the service of the doctor's view of the patient's best interests. This tradition was turned in an entirely new direction by a court case in 1957 that used the phrase "informed consent" for the first time in American jurisprudence.[15]

Through a series of court cases in the 1960s and 1970s and under the pressures of the cultural changes of the period, informed consent has reshaped the doctor–patient relationship. It has come to mean the negative right of patients to self-determination in medical matters; as such it represents a powerful expression of respect for the dignity of patients.

As the name suggests, informed consent embodies two important elements, one informational and one volitional. In the former aspect, informed consent requires that doctors supply patients with information, in terms they can understand, about their diagnosis and the risks and benefits associated with additional tests and treatments, including having none at all. Obviously, not everything a doctor knows about a disease and its treatment can be conveyed to every patient. Generally, doctors and patients are too unequal in knowledge to apply so high a standard. Therefore, the practical application of informed consent requires another standard, a definition of the scope of the doctor's duty to disclose.[16]

The first standard applied by courts was a professional standard. Doctors were obliged to disclose only what other competent doctors in their locality and specialty typically disclose to patients under similar circumstances. A significant moment in the evolution of informed consent was the court ruling in *Canterbury v. Spence,* in which the prevailing professional standard for interpreting the scope of disclosure was rejected.[17] The court applied a new standard, a reasonable person standard, that obliges doctors to disclose what patients need to know to make intelligent decisions. Although not all states have adopted the reasonable person standard explicitly, the cultural movement toward informed consent has been so overwhelming that even jurisdictions that still have a professional standard in law have a reasonable person standard in practice. The average competent doctor now reveals the full range of information patients need to make intelligent choices. Application of the professional standard has thus become identical to the reasonable person standard.

The Right to Refuse

The informational aspect of informed consent can be regarded as a positive right, a right of access to information. However, the larger cultural significance of informed consent is not in the sharing of information but in a relocation of decision-making authority. The most important feature of informed consent is the negative right of patients to refuse procedures by withholding or withdrawing consent. In general, competent patients can refuse any procedures offered by doctors, even those believed to be optimal, safe, and effective. Patients can choose alternatives or refuse treatment altogether.

The right to refuse at the heart of informed consent has been especially important in protecting the dignity of terminally ill patients. This right allows terminally ill patients to select ways of dying that avoid the use of measures they believe are extraordinary, that is, interventions that are futile or overly burdensome. In the 1970s and 1980s, this general movement of informed consent, especially in caring for the terminally ill, gave rise to advance directives.[18] These documents—living wills or durable powers of attorney—allow patients, while they are competent, to project their right to refuse into contexts in which incompetence is anticipated. In most cases, these are preemptive decisions to decline what are considered overly aggressive or simply unwanted medical procedures.

The larger cultural impact of the informed consent revolution has been to fix on the American scene a negative right that protects individuals from interference by doctors, other health care providers, or government. Even among nations that share the same general and medical culture as the United States, Americans have led the way in the legal and ethical development of informed consent.

It is easy to link this achievement to the value of respect for human dignity. On either religious or secular grounds, informed consent is an important protection of the special value of each individual person. On religious grounds, the right to refuse treatment, especially in the face of terminal illness, is an acknowledgment of each individual's authority to consult that person's own spiritual interpretation of the meaning of life and death and then use that framework to direct medical care. In the secular account, the inherent dignity of each person provides a basis for a right to self-determination. Alternately put, forcing patients to accept unwanted medical treatments imposes a meaning of life and is an objectification of a person, an act of treating a person like a thing. On either basis, therefore, informed consent establishes a characteristically American negative right, expressing the value of human dignity through a right of noninterference.

Freedom

Human dignity clearly provides a moral foundation for freedom. Views that persons have a spiritual nature or a civil inviolability (or both) protect a range of individual freedom. On religious grounds, persons have the liberty to live according to their own religious lights, an especially important liberty in a society of many religions. On secular grounds, persons have a right of noninterference, a right not to be dominated like a thing. Human dignity therefore entails individual freedom.

Individual freedom is also an independent value for Americans. The ideal of the free and independent citizen is immediately admirable to most Americans. Historical choices and political rhetoric shaped by this ideal have strongly influenced Americans' collective sense of self and have also affected the nation's conception of its role in world history. Self-reliance, individual initiative, and personal responsibility are strong themes throughout American culture. This emphasis on the individual is reinforced by an instinctive suspicion of and rebellion against rigid custom, regulation, and government. American distrust of government as both intrusive and inept is especially marked at the end of the twentieth century.[19] Americans are even ambiguous about intimate communities, feeling at once a need for the affective support of small towns, close friends, and families and at the same time a fear of their smothering control.

The history of the United States provides ample explanation for these attitudes. The ancestors of most Americans broke ties with comparatively homogeneous cultures, some by choice, some by force, most by the force of circumstances. They were uprooted from native communities and joined a culture in which community is largely an artifact built on the choices of individuals. Continued mobility toward frontiers and through internal migrations shows an ongoing willingness to separate from communities and to prize individual initiative. The defining moments of the birth of the nation—the War for Independence and the framing of the Constitution—were shaped by fear of government tyranny and a desire to protect individual liberty. The material successes of a comparatively free economy and the social mobility for many Americans that this free economy supported reinforced the value of individual liberty. Despite the multiple factors at play in every large historical event, the struggle for freedom is stressed constantly in Americans' understanding of the nation's development, from the Revolution to abolitionism, the Civil Rights Movement, and the liberation of women. Resistance to twentieth century totalitarianisms of the right and the left was justified on the same grounds. The growing cynicism at the end of the twentieth century about nearly all social institutions—government, the press, religion, the professions—has left little else in the field of values except those related to the individual and free choice. It is therefore no accident that Americans prize freedom.

The formal expression of this disposition in an ethical theory is libertarianism.[20] In this view, the dignity of the person makes individual liberty the highest value. Interference with liberty is justified only to prevent or redress violence or fraud, themselves fundamental interferences with liberty. For libertarians, all rights (except those linked to suppressing violence and fraud) are negative rights of noninterference. Positive rights, because they require government action with its attendant regulation and taxes, are rejected. Government action on behalf of claims for positive rights, generally efforts to secure access to needed goods and services, interferes with individual liberty and therefore violates persons' true rights, negative rights. Libertarians thus favor minimal government and maximal individual freedom, in many ways a quintessentially American stance.

Despite the genuine significance of freedom, especially as an expression of human dignity, this extreme ethical theory and the general American disposition that it captures is unacceptable.[21] To separate freedom from its link to human dignity and to put it forth as an absolute value misinterprets fundamental aspects of the human condition and leads to many troubling consequences.

Individualism and Equality

An extreme emphasis on freedom is nearly always linked to an excessive individualism that regards social organizations and communities as mere collections of individuals. Therefore, this view promotes selfishness and fosters loneliness and alienation. American inability or unwillingness to acknowledge that the production of healthy and independent individuals requires well-functioning social institutions, especially families and neighborhoods, lies behind much of the recent decline in these vital institutions. In short, individualism of this extreme kind underappreciates and undermines persons' social nature and the communities that compose it.[22]

Ironically, commitment to an absolutist theoretical model of freedom also frustrates efforts to build and expand freedom in practical terms. The right to education is a good example. Libertarian principles would recognize only a negative right of education, that is, noninterference with the efforts of adults to educate themselves and their children. Ideally, there would be no taxes for education, no government regulation, indeed, no public schools. Leaving people alone to educate themselves, however, would mean that some, perhaps many, would get little or no education. Theoretical insistence on freedom would have created a substantial practical loss of freedom. What kind of real freedom does an illiterate adult have in an information age?

This extreme degree of emphasis on individual freedom also threatens to undermine the theory of democratic decision-making. If even one person objects to a measure passed by the majority and has to live under a law not of his or her own choosing, freedom is violated; but to preserve all individual freedom from such an implication would mean chaos: rule by universal veto. Democracy is meaningless without both respect for individuals *and* a willingness to accept majority rule. Democracy, that is, cannot exist without social limitations on individual freedom.

Finally, the libertarian theory and strain in American culture represent a tyranny of just one value. Of course, freedom is a value and a very important one for Americans, but this theory and disposition place freedom permanently and in all situations above all other values. This is a radical revision of the moral pluralism at the heart of common sense. Multiple values have to be acknowledged and balanced, the details of concrete situations helping to determine which value or values have priority at a given time. Only extremists place one value consistently before all others.

One particular value that the libertarian view ignores is the other critical element in the value of human dignity: equality. All humans have equal moral dignity. An omnivorous conception of freedom makes the demands of respecting this value of equality impossible. This is especially obvious when government action is needed to establish or foster equality because government action always entails limits on someone's freedom through prohibitions, mandates, or taxes. There is no easy resolution of this tension at the heart of dignity, of the conflict between freedom and equality. It is clear, however, that both extremes are unacceptable. The demand for total equality without the constraint of individual freedom is a formula for tyranny. The demand for total individual freedom without commitment to equality is a formula for anarchy. Under both tyranny and anarchy, the strong prey on the weak. The

challenge of modern life is to strike a balance between the two values of freedom and equality, a balance that does justice to both aspects of human dignity. In practical terms, this means acknowledging some pragmatic combination of negative individual rights of noninterference and positive rights of equal
access to needed goods and services.

The Right to Health Care

The positive right at stake in health care—universal access to basic health
services—has a problematic standing among Americans. This right and its
ambiguous reception lie at the very heart of the health care reform debate.[23]
The link of this right to the value of human dignity is straightforward. Without regular access to health care, mortality and morbidity rates increase.
Consequently, human lives, lives that are each theoretically of absolute and
intrinsic value, are unnecessarily cut short and subjected to needless pain and
suffering. To acquiesce to this situation is to disvalue human dignity.

It is important to stress the moral limits of this insight. Although negative
rights forbid the harm of interference with freedoms, a positive right, such as
a right to health care, creates an obligation to provide benefits. An immediate problem, typical of positive rights, is one of scope. What kind and how
many benefits must be provided and at what cost to whom? Commitment to
human dignity does entail respect for the absolute and intrinsic value of each
person. However, it cannot entail a moral obligation to provide an open-ended
and potentially endless list of health care benefits to all persons. Such an
unbounded obligation would conflict with other obligations individuals have,
including obligations to themselves, and would lead to a view of persons as
merely resources for satisfying others' needs with no space left for personal
self-determination. It would overwhelm any conception of private discretionary use of time and resources. Moreover, such an open-ended health care
obligation would mean the inability to fund other important public priorities.

Therefore, theoretical limits on a positive right to health care are necessary if the claim for this right can have any chance for success in practice.
Like the right to education, a meaningful right to health care must be limited.
Some limits can be defined by appeal to the philosophical idea of a duty to
provide "easy rescue,"[24] according to which an individual is not obliged to
do everything possible to rescue another in peril, but only what can be done
easily, which is to say, without great danger or cost to the rescuer. Thus, for
example, a nonswimmer is not obliged to dive into a lake to attempt to save
a drowning person but is certainly obliged to throw a floatation device to the
victim or call for the help of a competent swimmer. The right to health care
must be similarly delimited. It cannot mean a right to every benefit that health

care can provide, but rather only a right to a reasonable package of benefits that can be afforded without great sacrifice by society as a whole.

The verbal formula sometimes used to capture this point is a *basic benefit package*. This is an important term, but one that is necessarily underdefined and vague.[25] Conceptual analysis of the notion of basic health care or a basic benefit package cannot reveal which medical procedures are included and which are not. Instead, what is basic must be determined by reference to a dynamic combination of individual need, the state of technology, the general economy, public expectations, and political realities. A useful starting point for a normative discussion of what basic coverage should include might begin with a description of what in fact operates as basic in the present situation. One might, for example, say that basic is what is included in a moderately priced insurance package available to middle income Americans. Clearly, this is the beginning of the discussion, not the end. In defining a basic benefit package for all Americans, adjustments may have to be made from this starting point, subtracting benefits too costly to provide for everyone and adding benefits as medical technologies and delivery systems evolve. Nonetheless, focusing on an average insurance package provides a meaningful and concrete starting point.

Also at stake in the debate about a right to health care are the other elements inevitably raised by a positive right, namely, government action and taxation. There is no reason to believe that the private health insurance industry or the health care marketplace operating on its own will be able to achieve universal access to health care. In fact, it was the evident failure of the marketplace to bring health care to the high-risk populations of the elderly and the poor that led to government action in the 1960s in the form of the Medicare and Medicaid programs. It is the evident failure of the marketplace to insure nearly 40 million Americans that provides part of the contemporary energy for reform. Present market pressures, however, favor cost containment, not expanded access.

Assuring universal access to health care will therefore require additional government action. Determining exactly what kinds and what extent of government action will require not only a delineation of individuals' rights, but also a prudential assessment of the benefits to be derived versus the burdens associated with the growth of bureaucracy and regulation. Amounts and kinds of new taxes must also be examined frankly because, regardless of potential savings, universal access means bringing into the system millions of Americans who are presently unable (and some unwilling) to pay the costs of their own care. It is impossible to determine in theory how much taxation is too much before health care reform would pass beyond the boundaries of the obligation of easy rescue. Every nation must consult its own history, needs, and resources. It is revealing, however, to note that every other nation in the world that has been influenced strongly by the Judeo–Christian religious tradition and the European Enlightenment has already created universal access for all its citizens. As a rule, these nations expect more government action and pay more taxes than Americans.[26]

Two Tiers

Another important dimension of the debate over the right to health care involves the impact of universal coverage on those who already have health insurance and those who in any system of coverage would be willing and able to buy additional benefits on their own. It might be argued that the absolute and intrinsic character of human dignity at the root of our political culture demands an equality of treatment in the health care arena. Certainly health care touches the existential equalities of human life—physical and mental illness and death itself—in more profound ways than most other activities. A strong argument can be made that equality is therefore more imperative here than in other areas of social life.[27]

Nevertheless, it appears obvious that American commitment to a wide range of individual self-determination and the political liberties that this entails must create limits on the amount of equality achievable in the health care arena. Inevitably, even were universal coverage achieved, at least two tiers of health care would still exist in the United States,[28] one composed of those who rely wholly on the publicly provided, subsidized, or mandated basic benefit package, and the other composed of those who buy out of or above this coverage. How these two tiers are structured can make all the difference between a morally tolerable, if less than ideal, situation and a morally intolerable one.

Suppose future health care reform results in a basic but comprehensive system of benefits that is mandated by the government and relied on exclusively by the great majority of Americans, say eighty to ninety percent. The remaining minority is willing and able to buy additional health care on their own. This would be a tolerable compromise between the equality and freedom at the heart of human dignity. Suppose, on the other hand, that the basic benefit package mandated under health reform is so minimal that only a minority of the least well-off Americans rely on it, and only because they cannot afford anything else. At the same time, the vast majority of Americans are willing and able to buy above this minimum. Under these circumstances, reform would have simply recreated welfare medicine. Such a system would support the reification of two different standards of care for patients. The lower-tier welfare program would be a political orphan, without popular support and chronically underfunded. Inevitably, its comprehensiveness and quality would suffer.

To achieve the first model and avoid the second, the basic benefit package of a reformed system will have to be more expansive—and expensive—than simply what is deemed minimally decent. It will have to be comprehensive enough to satisfy middle-class Americans. In short, the political strategy that advances the moral point here is to tie the interests of the poor who depend upon public support to the interests of the politically powerful middle class by creating a health care funding and delivery mechanism that both groups of Americans share and whose quality they are both concerned to maintain and enhance.

There are probably many systems of health care funding and delivery that are consistent with respect for human dignity, but it is becoming increasingly clear to many Americans that the barriers to care created by lack of insurance have created a situation incompatible with respect for human dignity. The challenge for the United States is to return to the task of crafting a conception of the right to health care that does justice to the special value of each person and fits with American political culture, especially with the marked disposition toward negative rights and individual freedom. Americans have led the world in the development of the negative human right of informed consent as an expression of human dignity. The United States now must grapple with the conflict between the legitimate demands for a positive right to health care and traditional anxieties about recognizing positive rights.

There is no evidence, historically or empirically, to believe that the marketplace operating on its own principles and motives is capable of creating a right to health care, of developing a system that provides health care basics to all. Moreover, if a basic amount of health care is a right of all Americans, the strategy of leaving initiatives in the arena to the states is inherently flawed. Progress toward realizing a right to health care requires leadership from the federal government, at least in managing markets and providing minimal standards for the states.

Unofficial Americans

There is a final vexing question of public policy raised by the moral imperative to create universal health coverage. Obviously, the argument for human dignity applies to all human beings, whether they are citizens of the United States or not. Nothing in the religious or secular arguments for dignity depends on citizenship in the United States or any other sort of citizenship. The establishment of the Judeo–Christian foundation for this position preceded the formation of the United States by centuries. A person has dignity on this account because of God, not because of country. Although the development of the secular foundation for dignity surrounded the framing of the Constitution and

Bill of Rights and in that context American citizenship was presumed, there is no firm secular link between fundamental rights and citizenship. By world standards, the United States has historically had permissive immigration and naturalization regulations that tend to erase strong distinctions between citizen and noncitizen. The U.S. courts have applied many basic constitutional rights to noncitizens living in the country. Moreover, the history of American action abroad and the political rhetoric supporting it indicates a strong national belief that fundamental rights are not American in origin or character but are human rights due to all persons in all nations.

However, the context of this argument for universal coverage is also plainly set within a given political community: the United States of America. Abstract values like respect for human dignity must be given concrete reality in a real community by virtue of the structure of mutual relationships, particularly in this case as defined by the rights and responsibilities of citizenship. The practical moral duty to create universal coverage that has been argued for here applies to Americans. Somalis and Guatemalans have human dignity as well and should have a right to basic health care; it is not clear, however, that the United States has a duty, at least not the same duty owed to its citizens, to provide health care to them. Furthermore, other nations' economies, cultures, and health care needs can be so different as to make conversation about an international basic benefit package nearly meaningless, except in the most abstract terms. If this point is granted, that Americans have duties regarding health care to other Americans but not (the same duties) to citizens in other nations, what is the situation with regard to citizens of other nations living illegally in the United States?[29]

Despite the unofficial status of these individuals and their families, there are good reasons to extend the goal of universal coverage to undocumented workers and their families. First, many children in these families are born in the United States and are therefore citizens. It would be both inhumane and foolish to cover a family's children with a basic package of health care while denying the same coverage to the children's parents, the very persons who are, after all, the primary health care providers for the children. Second, most of these individuals and their families are working and paying taxes and thus are supporting the nation's economy and social service structure by their taxes. In fact, their taxes help to pay for Medicare, Medicaid, and the tax advantages of those with private health insurance. Denying them health coverage would require them to continue to contribute to the nation's health care system while at the same time refusing to let them benefit from it. Finally, efforts to isolate noncitizens from citizens in the context of health care needs would not only create administrative difficulties, but would also sap the natural sympathetic responses of health care providers. Is the nation best served by doctors and nurses who can refuse to respond to the immediate sufferings of people because they are not (or may not be) American citizens? Can the nation's best interests lie in creating systematic delays in providing needed health care in order to certify citizenship?

Problems of immigration and the security of the nation's borders are large, complex, and well beyond the scope of this exploration. Certainly, it would not be prudent to create entitlements to health care irrespective of citizenship in ways that provide new incentives for illegal entry and residence in the United States. At the same time, it would be wrong and plainly incompatible with the spirit of the value of human dignity to deny the benefits of universal coverage to undocumented workers and their families who are living and working in the United States.

Notes

1. Gabriel Marcel, *The Existential Background of Human Dignity* (Cambridge, Mass.: Harvard University Press, 1963).
2. Beauchamp and Childress, *Principles of Biomedical Ethics*, pp. 120-188.
3. Jacques Maritain, *Man and the State* (Chicago: University of Chicago Press, 1956); and Jurgen Moltmann, *On Human Dignity: Political Theology and Ethics*, trans. Douglas Meeks (Philadelphia: Fortress Press, 1984).
4. Bellah et al., *Habits of the Heart*, pp. 237-249.
5. Immanuel Kant, *Grounding for the Metaphysics of Morals*, trans. James W. Ellington (Indianapolis, Ind.: Hackett Publishing Co, 1981), 35-44; and Wills, *Explaining America*.
6. See, e.g., Charles Fried, *Right and Wrong* (Cambridge, Mass.: Harvard University Press, 1978).
7. Edward Dumbauld, ed., *The Political Writings of Thomas Jefferson* (Indianapolis, Ind.: Bobbs-Merrill, 1955), ix.
8. Kant, *Grounding for the Metaphysics of Morals*, pp. 35-44.
9. See, generally, David Lyons, *Rights* (Belmont, California: Wadsworth Publishing Company, 1979).
10. On negative versus positive rights in health care, see Tom L. Beauchamp and Ruth R. Faden, "The Right to Health and the Right to Health Care," *Journal of Medicine and Philosophy* 4, (1979): 119-31.
11. The Sixth Amendment to the United States Constitution (in the Bill of Rights) reads: "In all criminal prosecutions, the accused shall enjoy the right to a speedy and public trial, by an impartial jury of the state and district wherein the crime shall have been committed, and to be informed of the nature and the cause of the accusation; to be confronted with the witnesses against him; to have compulsory process for obtaining witnesses in his favor, and to have the assistance of counsel for his defense.
12. David Tyack, *Law and the Shaping of Public Education* (Madison, Wisc.: University of Wisconsin Press, 1987).
13. A. H. Robertson, *Human Rights in Europe* (New York: Oceana Press, 1963).
14. See generally, Ruth R. Faden and Tom L. Beauchamp, *A History and Theory of Informed Consent* (New York: Oxford University Press, 1986).

15. The case was *Salgo v. Leland Stanford Jr. University Board of Trustees. Ibid.*, pp. 125-132.
16. Beauchamp and Childress, *Principles of Biomedical Ethics*, pp. 142-157.
17. *Canterbury v. Spence*, 464 F.2d 772 (1977).
18. L. Emmanuel, "Advance Directives: What Have We Learned So Far?" *Journal of Clinical Ethics* 4, no. 1 (1993): 8-16.
19. Blendon et al., *Health Affairs*, p. 284.
20. The philosophical case for libertarianism is laid out in Robert Nozick, *Anarchy, State, and Utopia* (New York: Basic Books, 1971).
21. Charles J. Dougherty, *American Health Care: Realities, Rights, and Reforms* (New York: Oxford University Press, 1988), 69-91.
22. Charles J. Dougherty, "The Excesses of Individualism," *Health Progress* 55, no. 1 (1992): 22-28.
23. Dougherty, *American Health Care*, pp. 23-34.
24. Beauchamp and Childress, *Principles of Biomedical Ethics*, pp. 266-67.
25. See, e.g., Robert Veatch, "What Counts as Basic Health Care? Private Values and Public Policy," *Hastings Center Report* 24, no. 3 (1994), 20-21.
26. "What the Taxman Takes," *The Economist* vol. 326, no. 7802 (March 13, 1993): 83-84.
27. Charles J. Dougherty, "Equality and Inequality in American Health Care," in *Freedom and Equality*, ed. Esther Mackintosh (Washington, D.C.: Federation of State Humanities Councils, 1992), 6-17.
28. Tristram Engelhardt, "Why a Two-tier System of Health Care Delivery is Morally Unavoidable," in *Rationing America's Medical Care: The Oregon Plan and Beyond*, ed. Martin Strosberg et al. (Washington, D.C.: Brookings Institution, 1992), 196-207.
29. K. Siddharthan and S. Alalasundaram, "Undocumented Aliens and Uncompensated Care: Whose Responsibility?" *American Journal of Public Health* 83, no. 3 (1993): 410-12.

4

Caring

Fiduciary Responsibilities

The health care system is a tremendous economic engine, consuming more than one of every seven dollars in the U.S. economy. It is a complex, often confusing bureaucracy that provides a wide array of services, from mammography to sports medicine, from heart transplantation to hospice. The financial and regulatory dimensions of the system are baroque. The scientific basis and technological power of modern health care interventions can be awesome. Within the space of two or perhaps three generations, the health care system has moved from a well-meaning but largely ineffectual network of altruistic providers to a complex industrial arrangement of professional and institutional providers who can extend lives and improve their quality through new technologies of curing and disease management.

Behind this daunting social reality stands a simple moral value that motivates the entire enterprise. Health care is grounded in caring.[1] It arises from a sympathetic response to the suffering of others. The humble fact of human frailty, of the inevitable brokenness and brevity of human life, shapes the range and depth of needs to which health care is a response. The rise of cosmetic health care interventions, elective surgery, and the whole range of new opportunities to create marginal improvements in health or function can easily disguise this fundamental fact. Health care arises in response to the vulnerability of persons to physical pain, mental suffering, loss of function, fear of death, and death itself. The hallmark of health care need, at its most basic level, is therefore human vulnerability.

Because such vulnerability is exceptionally easy to exploit—through false promises, quackery, financial manipulations—health care professionals take on special moral responsibilities to protect patients. This helps to account for why the Hippocratic oath is one of the earliest extant documents in the West that focuses on moral obligations.[2] Even in the ancient period, it was clear to the ancestors of today's doctors that health care service to patients meant managing vulnerability within a context of special professional responsibility. This insight forms the basis of the notion of fiduciary agency, a defining characteristic of a professional. A fiduciary agent, as the root of the name suggests, is one who acts out of a relationship of faithfulness (*fides*) with a client or patient.

The practical relevance of such faithfulness is the duty to place the interests of the client or patient first. This does not entail the fatuous notion that doctors, nurses, and others who are fiduciary agents have no self-interest, nor that it is unprofessional for them to make some decisions based on self-interest. Instead, the regulatory ideal of fiduciary agency requires health care professionals to place their patient's interests first whenever there is a real or possible conflict between that patient's interests and provider self-interest or the interests of other parties.[3] The obligation further entails a duty to avoid the creation of such conflicts. A doctor, for example, considering the appropriateness of a procedure for a patient may have an explicit conflict of interest because he or she benefits financially either by providing the treatment (as in the case of fee-for-service reimbursement) or by withholding the treatment (as in the case of capitated reimbursement). In such a circumstance, the doctor's first moral obligation is to decide the issue on the basis of the patient's interests first. Doctors and other health care professionals are also obliged to scrutinize the details of conflict-producing relationships, like reimbursement arrangements, in order to avoid potential conflicts or to soften their impact when conflicts are inevitable.

The duty to avoid the creation of conflicts also involves the question of appearances. In addition to resolving conflicts on behalf of patients' interests and avoiding creation of conflicts at the outset, professionals should avoid creating situations that provide an appearance of conflict. There is a deeper point here than merely preserving good public relations. From a moral perspective, patients must trust doctors before they can expose their vulnerability. The appearance of conflict can act as a barrier to persons needing care. Appearances alone, whether the conflict is real or not, can undermine the trust needed to establish and maintain effective doctor–patient relationships.

The importance of appearances is clear at two levels. The more obvious is the interpersonal. Individuals must trust their own doctors or else they will not seek their advice in times of need or follow their advice when they receive it. The public must also have a basic trust in health care professionals generally. In cases of medical need of any complexity, patients are referred from one health care professional to another. In serious cases, patients are treated by numerous doctors, nurses, and allied health professionals. Trusting one's own family doctor in such a circumstance is insufficient. In such contemporary therapeutic contexts, patients must have a readiness to trust virtually every health care professional encountered. The present system leaves little time for developing personal relationships with the numerous professionals involved in complex cases. Yet trust is still required for successful therapy. The public appearance of trustworthiness sets the stage for this.

Altruism

In addition to the obligation of fiduciary agency, which acts as a cognitive barrier against conflicts of interest, patient vulnerability is also protected by the affective stance of health professionals. In the immediacy of responding to the needs of patients, the concrete expression of fiduciary agency is more likely to be carried by the emotions of the professional than by any reflection on obligations. Agency means acting. From this point of view, it is far more important that a health care professional should *feel* a certain way about duty than it is that this professional should *think* a certain way about it. The natural altruism at the heart of health care, a sense of practical compassion for the sufferings of patients, is the central emotional bulwark protecting patient vulnerability.[4] The integration of both elements, of cognitive commitment to fiduciary agency and of the appropriate emotional altruism, fosters the creation of habits of feeling for and acting on behalf of patients. These habits constitute the core virtues of health care professionals.

The fact that need and vulnerability lie at the heart of the health care enterprise has been acknowledged at the social level by the historical understanding that health care institutions provide community services. In other terms, health care, although it must borrow many of the techniques of business, is not itself a business. Abuses abound, but most institutional providers of health care—hospitals, home health care agencies, and visiting nurses associations—regard themselves as committed primarily to a mission centered on service to community and individual needs.[5] Even when hospitals, nursing homes, and doctors' group practices are organized for profit, their sense of mission distinguishes them from the business world in general. Such mission commitments give rise in many cases to the provision of an array of special services provided to communities: free or subsidized health care for indigent patients, free or low-cost screening programs, health education efforts, programs to bring needed services into underserved areas, etc. This sense of mission and the charitable activities it often generates constitute the historical justification for the not-for-profit status of many of these providers.[6]

Foundations

Uniting the professional commitment to fiduciary responsibility and the personal and institutional altruism in health care is the value of care itself. Without a predisposition to care, the duty to be an agent who acts on behalf of another would make little sense. Without daily commitments to care, individual and group altruisms would have little effect. The moral value of care is expressed in both an attitude of caring *about* and a disciplined practice of caring *for*.[7]

Four elements of care can be distinguished.[8] First, care is attentive. It arises from a certain disciplined listening to needs, often those of others but not exclusively so. The opposite of the value of care is not hostility or hatred but indifference. Patients readily identify a caring health care professional as someone who listens, a caring institution as a place where their needs are the focus. Indifference, by contrast, is defined by routine, by unyielding rules, by a certain abstracting from the pathos of the context of need. It ignores, and therefore it remains in ignorance of the needs presented by the person in the examining room, the community across the neighborhood, the conscience inside.

Care is responsive. Whereas attentiveness requires passivity (though a focused and skilled passivity), care also demands action. Attentiveness is the origin of caring *about*; responsiveness the upshot of caring *for*. Real care is not sentimental and private, but energetic and other oriented. Arriving at the scene of a traffic accident, for example, those who only care *about* may be paralyzed with sympathy and grief. Those who care *for* move past their overwhelmed attentiveness and render practical assistance. Care is not content to listen: It acts.

Of course, care itself does not act; people who care act. So care is responsible. To care is to know that I must do this, and we must do that. Because a stance of indifference is always an option, those who care are volunteers. People cannot be conscripted into care (although they plainly can be conscripted into the work of care). The moral logic of voluntarism is evasive, yet familiar. Sometimes a person or an organization of persons just "knows" that this person or project is their responsibility. They step forward and care. Families who provide care for sick and dying loved ones often exhibit this element of responsibility, sometimes to heroic lengths.

Finally, care is competent. A person who wants to care must be able to care. Someone intent on care does not want to be inept or meddling. The response to need must be effective where possible but appropriate in every case. In health care, cure is often the explicitly desired goal of care, but competent care is always desirable as the medium when cure is possible and as the goal itself when cure is not possible.

These aspects of the value of care underscore some of the earlier points about morality in general. Like morality, care is emotion laden, not only in the sense that emotions can set the goals of moral conduct (easing others' pain, for example), but also in the deeper sense that emotions are part of the basis of morality (attending to the feelings of others, for example).[9] Like morality, care is situated; it must have a context, a subject, a goal. Like morality, care is practical. Its intent is to direct conduct, to make a difference.

Finally, like morality, care is social. It is predicated on the facts of need, attentiveness to need, and response to need. Thus, the value of care is incompatible with an extreme individualism and an exaggerated stress on autonomy. On the contrary, care can make sense only in a world of dependencies, a world in which vulnerable people depend on other people, relationships, and institutions to address their needs.

Mission and Margin

In the world of contemporary health care, caring about and caring for require professionals with fiduciary obligations and feelings of altruism placing the interests of their patients first and working in institutions with mission commitments that place service to the needs of communities above business interests. Whether such a simple picture has ever been wholly or even largely true is debatable.[10] Nevertheless, this image was an important regulative ideal that put brakes on the inevitable expression of self-interested behavior. Unfortunately, in contemporary American health care, these professional and institutional commitments to care—reality and image—are under exceptional pressure. The ideal of caring is losing its appeal and its ability to regulate professional and institutional behavior.

It is useful to restate that this inherited ideal did not imply monastic commitments on the part of professionals or hostility to business methods on the part of institutions. Health care professionals have served their own interests as they have served their patients. American doctors in particular have done exceptionally well for themselves in the second half of the twentieth century, especially after the introduction of Medicare. Despite large increases in their numbers, the average income of doctors, particularly specialists, has risen dramatically.[11] Although there is presently downward pressures on some specialists' income, most doctors will fare comparatively well into the foreseeable future.

Even the most dedicated, religiously committed American hospital employs all the business techniques of the contemporary corporation, including those of billing and collection, to ensure a positive margin, if not a profit in the technical sense. This point is captured in a cliché well known in not-for-profit hospital circles: "No margin, no mission."[12] Many hospitals have done exceptionally well in the former category.

In spite of these admissions, the fact remains that for most health care professionals in the United States in this century and for most of the institutions in which they work, the self-interest that is assumed to drive contemporary business has been held at arms length. Business techniques were adopted as the *means* by which the goals of service to individual patients and to communities were pursued. The business aspects of health care professionals and institutions were not considered ends in themselves. The aim was mission, not margin. This is a stronger point than the defense often given for capitalism, namely, that the community is served indirectly when everyone seeks their own interest directly. Businesses pursing their own margins directly produce the jobs and wealth that serve the whole community indirectly. In contrast, for the most part, doctors and hospitals have sought to serve the interests of patients and communities *directly*.

This same point can be made using the concept of commodity.[13] An object or service that is produced for the sake of the profit that it can generate is a commodity. The world of business is constituted by the production and exchange of commodities. Traditionally, health care stood outside the business world because health services were not viewed as commodities. These services were not developed or delivered for the sake of making money, even though money was the necessary medium for their development and delivery. Because of this difference, some of the more egregious aspects of business were rejected by health care professionals and institutions.[14] For most of this century, for example, professional associations prohibited advertisement by their members, and local medical associations reined in their colleagues' overcharging by professional persuasion. Price was not to be determined by what the market could bear, but by a sense of the customary. Traditionally, hospitals were not places to make money. One of the legal constraints of a not-for-profit hospital, for example, is that whatever surplus it generates must be reinvested into the hospital itself. Surplus cannot be distributed as profit to owners or investors.[15]

New Pressures

The last quarter of the twentieth century has seen the beginnings of dramatic changes on these counts. The United States Supreme Court ruling in the *Goldfarb v. Virginia State Bar* case in 1975 barred professional organizations, including medical associations, from prohibiting their members from advertising.[16] Doctors now advertise freely and ubiquitously. Increasingly, doctors are becoming employees of hospitals, physician–hospital organizations, HMOs, and other kinds of delivery networks.[17] Many of these organizations are for-profit entities. Investor-owned for-profit hospitals, nursing homes, and home health care agencies have spread throughout the American scene. Pressures to cut costs by avoiding hospitalization in a context of overcapacity has generated extremes of competitive behavior in the hospital sector. Increased competition between hospitals has led to behavior on the part of many not-for-profit organizations that makes them difficult to distinguish from their for-profit cousins.

Other factors have heightened the business aspects of health care. The excess of medical specialists and of hospital beds has set the stage for intense competition for patients. At the same time, consumers, insurance companies, and employers are demanding more efficiency and new cost-containing measures that are themselves exacerbating competitive pressures and leading to new business combinations. The widespread sense that Americans have reached fiscal and political limitations in health care spending has led to the search for new sources of funds for research and development and for capital investment, frequently from business investors expecting short-term profits.[18] The impact of graduate medical education, the scrutiny of accrediting agencies, heightened awareness of legal liability, increased public expectations, and the diffusion of medical technology and expertise have led to a general homogenization of American health care. Although significant differences in regional practice styles persist, uniformly high quality of care across America's hospitals has erased or softened traditional distinctions between religious and nonreligious hospitals, public and private hospitals, profit and not-for-profit hospitals, secondary and tertiary care hospitals,[19] causing many hospitals to lose their economic niches in the health care economy, thereby increasing competitive pressures throughout the system.

At the same time that these competitive phenomena are in the ascendancy, a consumer revolution in health care comprising greater public access to health-related information, the institutionalization of informed consent, and performance scorecards for providers has defeated the traditional medical paternalism. The shadow side of this success story lies in what may have been lost with the rejected paternalism. The *noblesse oblige* characteristic of medical paternalism was closely linked to many aspects of professional caring,

especially to compassion and "going the extra mile."[20] In the new world of
the doctor–patient relationship, the patient is no longer a child in relationship to a health provider/parent; rather, the relationship is now adult to adult.
In most respects, this change is welcome. It has resolved many of the abuses
typical of the former paternalism.

Nevertheless, this change has brought new challenges into therapeutic
relationships. Under the older model, it was easier to understand why doctors, nurses, or other health care professionals had special obligations to their
patients, over and above their general moral obligations to other persons. They
were professionals caring for patients. If contemporary therapeutic relationships are truly adult to adult and shaped by the patient's right to informed
consent, professionals may come to feel less professional and more like ordinary business people. Doctors are certainly feeling less inhibited about their
own self-interests.[21] Put in other terms, there is a general movement away
from a doctor–patient relationship that may have been aptly characterized as
covenantal, even feudal, toward one that is contractual. The hallmark of contract is an explicit mutual understanding of *quid pro quo*. If this is so, the
self-interest of the health care professional need not be submerged or always
placed second, certainly not if the patient is an adult who is informed of the
providers' self-interest and elects to proceed despite (or because of) it. In short,
some elements of the doctor–patient relationship that were characteristically
professional have become far more explicitly businesslike, with uncertain but
worrisome consequences.

On Doctors

In some respects, these movements may bring good things. Certainly, the older
model shielded considerable hypocrisy and cant; but there are reasons for
concern as well. Chief among them is the fear that heightened candor about
professional self-interest and freedom to act on it along with increased business and profit-driven behavior on the part of hospitals and other provider
networks will tend to drive out the caring dimension of health care.

The pressures mounting against contemporary doctors' ability and readiness to care are significant and troubling. Earlier generations of American
doctors practiced with a certain hauteur with respect to economics. Their
professional concern was their patients' best interests, and the costs of the
tests and treatments they ordered were literally someone else's business. This
attitude was reinforced by the spread of health insurance, especially first-dollar
coverage, that insulated both doctor and patient from cost considerations in
therapeutic contexts. A new world dawned in the late 1970s with the first
round of cost-related monitoring of doctors' professional activity, followed

by the introduction of Medicare's prospective payment or DRG (Diagnosis-Related Groups) system in the mid-1980s and by the frenetic spread of capitation and provider networks in the 1990s. Doctors now face an intimidating array of cost-related considerations, even barriers, to their professional efforts on behalf of patients.[22] Doctors must seek approval for most hospitalizations and are pressured to limit their patients' length of stay. Referral to specialists has been made more difficult. Doctors are subject to retrospective and even real-time review of charts for the financial appropriateness of their decision-making.

The spread of capitation raises its own moral issues. In many capitated plans, doctors are subcapitated so that they receive a fee per member per month whether they provide any services for the enrollee or not. This creates the central moral problem of capitation, namely, a financial incentive to under-treat.[23] Capitated doctors' revenue is set, regardless of whether services are provided. The provision of services increases expenses. Therefore, given a weakened sense of professional obligation, an economically motivated doctor will be inclined to do less. This perverse incentive, the opposite of the equally perverse fee-for-service incentive to overtreat, is made even worse in some situations by financial arrangements governing enrollee hospitalization and specialty care.[24] In a typical arrangement, doctors have access to two pools of money to cover the costs of these patient needs. The cost of each of their patients' hospitalization and every visit to a specialist is charged against these accounts. At the end of the fiscal period, all or some of the money not spent on hospitalization and specialty care can be kept by the doctor, thus creating a powerful financial incentive to minimize hospitalization and specialty care. It also creates a serious conflict of interest for this "gatekeeper"; every choice to hospitalize or refer to a specialist costs the doctor money.[25]

The impact of all these changes on the American medical profession has been serious. Many doctors are demoralized. They have lost a range of previously enjoyed professional autonomy,[26] and are subject to the scrutiny and regulation of a host of others, including nonprofessionals. Many doctors report that they would not choose to enter the profession again, nor would they advise others to do so. As a group, they have little confidence in solutions offered either by government or by the marketplace, especially when marketplace solutions are led by insurers.[27] The number of doctors who have sought shelter from these forces by becoming employees of hospitals or integrated delivery networks has increased with uncertain consequences. This demoralization of doctors, shared to some extent by nurses and other health care professionals, is plainly bad for these professionals, but it is also bad for the patients whom they serve. As indications of professional burnout increase, the pressures against caring mount: time, money, and regulation pressures. As these pressures increase, the personal core of the health care delivery system may be undermined. The least that can be said is that the doctor–patient relationship is undergoing dramatic and unprecedented changes. There is abundant experience worldwide for appreciating the challenges that face the medical profession when government is the financial master, but there are no models for this kind of marketplace domination.

The ability and willingness of health care professionals to discharge their traditional fiduciary duties to patients and to feel professional altruism are at stake. Without attention to this phenomenon, the changing health care environment may well produce a new generation of health care professionals who simply do not consider caring to be a fundamental part of their relationships with patients and do not feel the feelings required to make caring a reality in those relationships.

On Hospitals

Similar points can be made about the need to protect caring in health care institutions, especially in hospitals and the delivery networks into which they are evolving. Even if health care reform efforts were to succeed in achieving universal coverage, it is unlikely that any system of health insurance could ever be universal enough. Some people will always "fall through the cracks"— perhaps undocumented workers or foreign tourists or the homeless. The mission commitments of hospitals will have to be relied on to find ways to serve these individuals. Even if coverage were to become literally universal (perhaps through a payer of last resort for all uncovered patients), there would still be challenges for hospitals that will require a strong sense of mission. For example, unless there were serious risk adjustments in the reimbursement system, adjustments that would send more dollars to providers caring for the sicker and higher-risk populations, there will be need for institutions with a distinctive sense of mission, institutions that could place community needs above bottom-line interests. Some patients and some enrolled populations in networks will plainly be more profitable than others.[28] Persons likely to be among the least profitable, given the present character of American society, will also be marginalized in other ways: by race, ethnic status, and socioeconomic standing, for example. Communities will need institutions ready and willing to serve these populations. There will always be patients with diseases and conditions of decline who are especially difficult to care for, such as HIV and AIDS patients, those with drug-resistant tuberculosis, many psychiatric patients, and those in hospice care, who must be treated by professionals and institutions with special dedication that routinely goes beyond the range of "business as usual." Such morally outstanding professionals and institutions will always be needed.

Suppositions about universal coverage, however, are just that. For the fore-seeable future, millions of Americans will remain uninsured. They will rely for their care on hospitals that are ready and willing to provide uncompensated care. Such an institutional commitment appears increasingly heroic, even self-sacrificial, in the present environment of increased market competition and cuts in Medicare and Medicaid. Institutions that provide large amounts of uncompensated care may face the ultimate penalty of economic rationalization: closure. Competitive business models cannot be used to solve this problem. No one competes for patients who cannot pay. Solution of the problem of the uninsured can come only by way of government leadership, acting no doubt with the private and voluntary sectors but led inevitably by the federal government.

It is also important to remember that even providing garden-variety health care services to average American populations who have insurance still involves important encounters with vulnerability. Wholesale adoption of a business worldview is insufficient to protect these vulnerabilities. Patients and their families simply cannot be effective shoppers and consumers under conditions of pain, suffering, loss of function, and fear of death. "Let the buyer beware" may operate as an effective governing rule for the purchase of automobiles and refrigerators, although even here there is a clear role for government regulation to ensure the safety of individuals and the environment, but "let the buyer beware" can hardly suffice for appendectomies and dialysis.[29] Even if most American health care institutions adopt models and behaviors from the world of business, that is, even if most were to become organized for profit, it is important that these accretions from the world of business not be allowed to subvert dedication to mission and orientation to community service.

Protecting Care

What options are available for protecting care in the context of a rapidly chang-ing health care system? Several strategies suggest themselves. First, among the most broken parts of the contemporary system is the lack of a primary health care network. Too often, patients enter the system at inappropriate sites; many enter through hospital emergency rooms, for example. They miss opportunities for health promotion, prevention, and screening because they do not have a regular source of comprehensive and timely care. In addition to achieving universal health insurance coverage, one of the goals of genuine health care reform should be guaranteeing that every American is in some kind of structured health care network based on primary care.[30]

However, these primary care plans differ in other respects; a common de-nominator should be a care manager, an individual who is assigned to each patient and enrollee in the plan and who acts as their personal point of entry to the health care system. In many cases this role will be played by a doctor in family practice, pediatrics, general internal medicine, or obstetrics and gynecology. In other cases, physicians' assistants, nurse practitioners, or social workers may be the appropriate professionals. In any case, every American should know the name and the face of some individual to call in times of health care need. This contact can act as a patient advocate to secure the best possible array of services from the health care plan involved. Whether a doctor or not, the care manager can bear the mantel of the fiduciary obligation to act for the patient's best interest and to do so in a compassionate and sympathetic manner. Moreover, this person could be charged with integrating the whole array of services, from prevention to acute care to hospice, for the patients and enrollees that the plan serves. An arrangement of this sort would ensure that future networks remain patient centered and personal and that they protect the cognitive and affective commitments traditionally central to health care.

Second, professional space must be carved out for doctors to protect their own autonomy of practice and to end the oppressive micromanagement that has accumulated over the last generation. This will likely require the use of at least two mechanisms. Despite the traditional reluctance about government involvement, the need to contain rising health care costs will dictate that some kind of global budgeting be introduced into the system at the national level, iterated at the state level, and reiterated at the level of local health care plans.[31] Budgeting of this sort sets a limit on the amount of dollars available for a given period of time and challenges doctors and others working with them to create strategies for the efficient use of the money available for that period. In essence, the discipline of a national budget provokes grass-roots planning. By contrast, the present open-ended character of many reimbursement systems leaves few methods for containing costs except for increasingly detailed inspection of particular choices by particular doctors. Insurers determine who can be hospitalized. Network policies dictate access to specialists. Home health agencies shape the range of available therapies. Doctors have less and less clinical control, individually or professionally. Obviously, adopting global budgets and involving doctors in planning will require a role for government and a financial integration of the system beyond anything Americans are likely to support today. The alternative to government, however, is the market. Doctors are just beginning to experience the consequences of choosing this alternative.

In addition to effective global budgeting, doctors need far more developed and useful practice protocols or critical pathways.[32] These clinical guidelines would provide the broad outlines of standard responses to typical health care needs, with a defined range of discretion for clinicians. They would also create a legal presumption in favor of doctors when the guidelines are followed and therefore provide something of a safe haven against liability concerns. Most importantly, practice protocols would provide a professional defense of quality standards against ruthless cost cutters. In the past, doctors have rejected practice protocols as "cookie-cutter" medicine. In the future, they may look to them as their best defense against bottom-line–oriented network administrators.

If the trend toward employment of doctors in large delivery networks continues, steps must be taken to ensure that these professional employees have the ability to control elements of the health care delivery environment in ways that go beyond what is typically the authority of employees. In other words, some compromise must be reached between the traditional prerogatives of a professional and the status of an employee so that patients' interests can be protected by the medical profession's traditional commitments. In particular, the *real* ability of doctors to refer patients to hospitals and specialists outside their employment network must be protected.

Another arena for careful assessment of changes in the health care system involves the competition between health care plans, especially between hospitals. Most American hospitals have begun to contract, to downsize. Many have closed and more will do so.[33] Competition between hospitals will increase as they struggle to survive. In the long run, downsizing and closures may serve the interests of society as a whole. Many communities are significantly overbedded and would profit from having fewer beds and fewer hospitals. However, the competitive corporate behavior these strong pressures engender is not only wasteful economically, but also corrosive of the value of caring. At the same time that these competitive forces are rationalizing the hospital sector, serious regional planning must begin with an eye toward minimizing the ravages of competition. Planning should also aim at ensuring that inner cities and rural areas are not further disadvantaged by loss of their already fragile infrastructure. Explicit focus on the effects of competition in a planning process may also provide an opportunity to blunt some of the more extreme corporate behaviors that are incompatible with hospitals' traditional sense of mission and commitment to community service.

Intangibles

No patient or potential patient is safe if the language of care and caring drops out of public discourse about the changes occurring in health care and about the future of the system. Caring is especially vulnerable in the present economic environment because a great deal of caring is intangible and therefore not quantifiable. As money gets tighter and pressures to reduce costs increase, things and activities that can be easily counted may squeeze out concern for intangibles. To prevent this, ways must be found to count some of the phenomena associated with caring (especially consumer satisfaction) and the prerequisites of caring (especially time spent with patients and professional-to-patient ratios). Above all, health care planners and those attempting to renew health care reform must recover the language of caring and speak it without embarrassment, insisting that care be recognized as a core value at the heart of health care. Unless this happens, health care change will not amount to health care reform. Instead, it will be an evolution toward a highly efficient, economically lean system of health service delivery that may produce good outcomes for many people but that cares about neither the persons nor the communities it serves.

It is worth recalling periodically that despite all the advances in health care and its delivery, there is one inevitable, bad outcome for each of us, and no amount of health care, no type of health care reform can make any difference on this final score. Health care can extend life and avoid premature death. It can often produce important differences in the quality of life, but each of us must die; neither health care nor health care reform can cure the human condition. Health care can make a significant difference, however, in how we relate to one another through the years that each of us has. A reformed system of health care *may* improve delivery and health status. It *must* ensure that Americans care about and for one another through the special vulnerabilities of the human condition.

Notes

1. On caring, see M. Leininger, ed. *Caring: An Essential Need* (Thorofare, N.J.: Charles Stack, 1981).
2. See generally, Owsei Temkin and Lilian Temkin, eds., *Ancient Medicine* (Baltimore: Johns Hopkins University Press, 1967).
3. Eli Ginzberg, "Health Care and the Economy—A Conflict of Interests?" *The New England Journal of Medicine* 326, no. 1 (1992): 72-74; and Arnold Relman, "What Market Values are Doing to Medicine," *The Atlantic Monthly* vol. 269, no. 3 (March 1992): 99-106.
4. For a philosophical treatment of altruism, see Thomas Nagel, *The Possibility of Altruism* (Oxford: Clarendon Press, 1970).
5. On the history of American hospitals, see Rosemary Stevens, *In Sickness and in Wealth: American Hospitals in the Twentieth Century* (New York: Basic Books, 1989).
6. John O'Donnell and James H. Taylor, "The Bounds of Charity," *The New England Journal of Medicine*, 322, no. 1 (1990): 65-68.
7. Joan C. Tronto, *Moral Boundaries* (New York: Routledge, Chapman, and Hall, 1993), 101-10.

8. Tronto, *Moral Boundaries*, pp. 126–137.
9. Virginia Held, *Feminist Morality* (Chicago: University of Chicago Press, 1993), 52.
10. For a critical historical overview, see Paul Starr, *The Social Transformation of American Medicine* (New York: Basic Books, 1982).
11. Altman and Rosenthal, *New York Times* (Feb. 18, 1990), p. 20.
12. See, e.g., B. Blackwell, "A Piece of My Mind; No Margin, No Mission," *JAMA* 271, no. 19 (1994): 1466.
13. Charles J. Dougherty, "The Costs of Commercial Medicine," *Theoretical Medicine*, 11 (1990): 275–86.
14. Generally, see, Lawrence Nelson et al., "Taking the Train to a World of Strangers: Health Care Marketing and Ethics," *Hastings Center Report* 19, no. 4 (1989): 36–43.
15. O'Donnell and Taylor, "The Bounds of Charity," pp. 65–68.
16. Allen Dyer, "Ethics, Advertizing, and the Definition of a Profession," *Journal of Medical Ethics* 11, no. 2 (June 1985): 72–78.
17. J. Ludden, "Doctors as Employees," *Health Management Quarterly* 15, no. 1 (1993): 7–11.
18. See, e.g., Daniel Callahan, *Setting Limits* (New York: Simon and Schuster, 1987).
19. Ginzburg, *The Road to Reform*, pp. 21–39.
20. Marc Siegler, "A Right to Health Care: Ambiguity, Profesional Responsibility, and Patient Liberty," *Journal of Medicine and Philosophy* 4, no. 2 (1979): 148–56.
21. See, generally, George Agich, "Medicine as Business and Profession," *Theoretical Medicine* 11, no. 4 (1990): 311–24; and Charles J. Dougherty, "The Costs of Commercial Medicine," *Theoretical Medicine* 11, no. 4 (1990): 275–86.
22. F. Tingley, "The Use of Guidelines to Reduce Costs and Improve Quality: A Perspective from the Insurers," *Joint Commission Journal on Quality Improvement* 19, no. 8 (1993): 330–34; and L. Brown, "Political Evolution of Federal Health Care Regulation," *Health Affairs* 11, no. 4 (1992): 17–37.
23. Dougherty, *American Health Care*, pp. 153–57.
24. Eckholm, *New York Times*, p. 22.
25. Marc A. Rodwin, "Conflicts in Managed Care," *The New England Journal of Medicine* 332, no. 9 (1995): 604–607.
26. Eckholm, *New York Times*, p. 22.
27. Robert Blendon et al., "Health System Reform: Physicians' View on Critical Issues," *JAMA* 272, no. 19 (1994): 1546–50.
28. *Ibid*.
29. Dougherty, *American Health Care*, pp. 135–147.
30. Peter Franks, Paul Nutting, and Carolyn Clancy, "Health Care Reform, Primary Care, and the Need for Research," *JAMA* 270, no. 12 (1993):1449–53; and P. Budetti, "Achieving a Uniform Federal Primary Care Policy: Opportunities Presented by National Health Reform," *JAMA* 269, No. 4 (1993): 498–501.
31. Patricia Wolfe and Donald Moran, "Global Budgeting in the OECD Countries," *Health Care Financing Review* 14, no. 3 (1993): 55–76.
32. See, e.g., M. McClellan and R. Brooks, "Appropriateness of Care: A Comparison

of Global Budgets and Outcome Methods to Set Standards," *Medical Care* 30, no. 7 (1992): 565-86.

33. See, e.g., N. McKay and J. Coventry, "Rural Hospital Closures," *Medical Care* 31, no. 2 (1993): 130-40; and J. Dailey, H. Teter, and R. Cowley, "Trauma Center Closures: a National Assessment," *Journal of Trauma* 33, no. 4 (1992): 539-46.

5

Protection of the Least Well-off

Foundations

One of the most primitive of moral positions is self-love. In a sense this position is built into human bodies and psyches in the obvious fact that all persons first and foremost feel their own pain and pleasure, happiness and sorrow. People sometimes choose for others but always in the first case for themselves, although not always in a selfish fashion. No matter how public the moment or activity, there is an irreducible element of the personal that characterizes everyone's own experience.

However, morality requires a broader focus. It demands a movement of perspective from the most particular (me) to the less particular (my family, my tribe) toward the universal (my kind, my world). Yet even for those who espouse an explicitly universal ethic—the human species, for example—the daily realities of morality demand loyalty to particularities. Each of us has certain people to whom special responsibilities are owed, family, friends, and co-workers, for example. These particular responsibilities cannot be respected through a general commitment to humankind. In fact, such particular and general goals are often in conflict: the rural doctor on call for

the whole county also has a family that demands attention, the weekend acti-
vist for international refugee relief has other job responsibilities during the
week, the Habitat for Humanity volunteer must also repair his or her own
house. In fact, many ethicists have argued that such particular duties are more
morally binding than abstract commitments, that, for example, the person who
neglects his or her own children working for the children of the world has
inverted the proper order of obligations.[1]

Although valid, these observations may prove too much. Certainly, people
can fail morally by placing abstract commitments ahead of concrete duties,
but the dynamic of moral development plainly suggests the importance of
movement from the most particular (the self) toward the more universal.
Furthermore, a sense of obligation that moves beyond known parties to embrace concern for unknown others, especially needy strangers, is clearly a
prized element of morality. The story of the Good Samaritan, for example,
captures a central moral insight of the Judeo–Christian tradition. If moral obligation does originate with the self and have a proper link to particular relationships, how can obligation proceed beyond these limits toward greater
universality? How can morality capture the Good Samaritan insight, this intuitively obvious part of moral common sense?

The answer may be found in the contexts that create special moral duties,
duties not to everyone in general, but to this person or set of persons.[2] People
may be said to owe others special moral obligations in four ways: through
kindred relationships, voluntary assumption of duty, reciprocity, and special
need. People owe special obligations to their family members. When people
choose to come to another's aid, they voluntarily take on duties. People owe
duties to those who have benefitted or aided them. Finally, people owe duties
to those in special need: a person who collapses on the street, a flood victim,
someone overcome with anxiety.

Though this accounting of the sources of particular moral obligations appears to generate a very disparate list, there is a common theme. Each duty is
structured to protect a special vulnerability or dependence. Family members
depend on each other in myriad and intimate ways. A voluntary act of aid
without a sense of duty may leave the rescued individual worse off, abandoned,
for example, or treated without due care. Rendering aid creates a presumption of reciprocity; "one good turn deserves another." Because this is so, failure to return assistance to another who has been helpful can create vulnerability. The latter may be led to the false belief, for example, that the former
can be counted on. The case of special need involves vulnerability in a straightforward way.

The conclusion suggested by this common root of moral obligation is that
an affirmative response to protect others from vulnerability may be the primary moral mechanism that leads individuals from their own narrow concerns

into special moral relationships with others. Protection of vulnerability may be the moral motive that moves duty from focusing on the particular self toward concern for concrete others. It may be the same motive that drives morality toward universality, toward concern for anyone's vulnerability. If so, then protection of the most vulnerable, those least well-off, should be an especially powerful moral value.

Special Rights

This same point can be captured in the language of dignity and rights. Human dignity provides the grounds for a claim of universal and equal human rights. No person has more or less human dignity, an estimate of worth that is incalculably great in every case. Hence dignity is the basis at once for the special value placed on each individual and for the moral equality of all persons.

From this perspective, all human rights are the same. In addition to equal human rights, however, special rights are and ought to be recognized in special situations. Special rights, by law and by custom, are introduced into circumstances of marked inequality as a practical means of restoring or preserving equality. Children have rights that parents do not enjoy, students have rights that teachers do not have, and prisoners have rights that their jailers do not have. Children, students, and prisoners have these rights because members of these groups are so easily exploited in relations with parents, teachers, and jailers. The point is not that individuals in these groups have different standing as persons. They do not have more human rights. Rather, circumstances of unequal authority, knowledge, and power require special rights on the part of the more vulnerable party to ensure equality. Because of the general correlativity of rights and duties—one person's right creates another person's duty—parents, teachers, and jailers have special obligations in their relationships that correspond to the special rights of children, students, and prisoners.

This same point holds for patients. Doctors and other health care professionals have special obligations to patients, primarily a fiduciary responsibility to put the interests of their patients first. Corresponding to that duty are special rights on the part of patients. Hospital patients have special rights, for another example, rights not held by hospital administrators or by the doctors and nurses who work in hospitals.[3] Once again, these are not human rights in the most basic sense, but equalizing special rights designed to restore the balance inherent to universal human rights in characteristically unbalanced situations.

This point can be generalized and applied to any group that suffers a significant disadvantage in its relationship with others. Individuals have rights against society because of the graphic inequality between the individual and the group; this is especially clear in legal contexts. In criminal cases, for example, charges are expressed as the *United States versus Jane Smith* or the *People of the Commonwealth of Pennsylvania against Richard Jones*. Similarly, one can speak of minorities as having certain rights against the majority, rights designed to ensure protection in their vulnerable situation. Human rights protect our general vulnerabilities; special rights protect special vulnerabilities. The moral drive to protect the most vulnerable should thus be expressed as acknowledgment of their special rights.

Health Disparities

Some of the most marked vulnerabilities of people arise from the inequalities created by health status.[4] Some persons are born free of genetically inherited illness; others' genes doom or disable them from the start. Some are born into conditions supportive of healthy growth and development; others are thwarted by their surroundings. Some live and work in relatively safe conditions; others are subject to high rates of accident and injury. As a result of these differences, many Americans enjoy long, healthy lives; others have shorter life spans and greater morbidity.

The facts of these inequalities alone would be challenging enough to a moral framework committed to the equality inherent in human dignity, but other contemporary realities in the United States make the situation more challenging yet. Disproportionate suffering from high mortality and morbidity rates are linked systematically to other inequalities on the American scene.[5] Race, ethnicity, general socioeconomic status, and level of education are highly correlated with states of health. As a general rule, membership in a minority race or ethnic group, low socioeconomic standing, and fewer years of formal education create a strong likelihood of increased morbidity and shortened life span.

Not all the specific linkages involved are known; some that are known to some degree are not known clearly. Much remains to be learned, for example, about the power of genetic inheritance and the racial and ethnic factors at stake in that inheritance. It is not inconceivable that some of the racial and ethnic disparities in average birth weight or rates of hypertension may have a genetic basis or component. Yet some linkages are obvious even to the casual observer. It is very clear that minority racial and ethnic status overlaps in many cases with low socioeconomic status and fewer years of formal education. This means that whatever genetic factors may be involved in racial or ethnic health deficits, their effects are exaggerated by poverty and lack of education.

There are multiple links between poverty and illness, causation running both ways.[6] People living in poverty have less healthy diets, live in more polluted and dangerous surroundings (including areas with high levels of crime and street violence), have higher rates of many of the lifestyles and behaviors that trigger disease, and face substantial barriers in accessing timely and comprehensive health care. Lack of education can mean less knowledge about the prevention and causes of disease and less sophistication about the appropriate use of the health care system. Even where the relevant knowledge is available, poverty conspires against the ability to defer gratification. It encourages living for the moment because the future promises so little. This disposition militates against prevention and the development of positive health habits.

Many of these disadvantaging conditions can be traced more or less to racism and ethnic prejudice. Generations of slavery of African–Americans, for example, places this group at a unique disadvantage. Despite efforts of many to overcome racism, skin color remains a powerful trigger for prejudice throughout the United States. Continued prejudice based on ethnicity or linguistic and cultural differences certainly shapes the social conditions that affect the health status of many minority groups. There can be little doubt, for example, that bias against minorities accounts in part for the high rates of unemployment typical of minority communities.[7] High unemployment itself contributes to diminished health status through the other conditions it produces: poverty, drug and alcohol abuse, street crime, domestic violence, family disintegration, homelessness, and hopelessness.[8] It may be overly simple but not inaccurate to conclude that present inequalities in health status among racial and ethnic minorities are directly related to the relative poverty of their socioeconomic circumstances, which is itself linked to racial and ethnic prejudice in American life. Even admitting a role for genetic chance and a range of personal and social responsibilities, one clear line of causation of health-related inequality is rooted in a morally shameful dimension of America's past and present social realities.

Others fall into categories of exceptional vulnerability in health terms for reasons that are less clear. There has been an appalling increase in homelessness over the last several decades.[9] Since the mid-1960s, the proportion of public spending for children has declined while that for the elderly has increased.[10] Now the elderly are among the least poor of the age cohorts in the United States, whereas children are among the poorest. The frail elderly and those of any age who must rely on home assistance or institutional care continue to suffer for want of a rational long-term care system. Those with chronic mental illnesses are also among the most vulnerable. These Americans, along with members of minority racial and ethnic groups suffering from high rates of morbidity and mortality, are candidates for special rights designed to counterbalance the inequalities that they experience.

Religious Views

Put in terms of rights and duties, special rights for the least well-off create obligations on the part of relatively healthy, well-off Americans to design a system that takes the former's needs into consideration. The value of human dignity demands it.

Special concern for those who are least well-off can also be understood as a value in itself. Historically, Judeo–Christian societies have pointed with pride to special institutions and personal sacrifices made on behalf of the least well-off. There is more than one injunction in the Bible to the effect that a society is judged by how it cares for those least able to care for themselves.[11] Christianity has multiple historical links to the least well-off. It was born in the modest circumstances of its founder, became noteworthy (in part) because of the miraculous cures of some of the least well-off, and spread rapidly in its early years among the poor and among slaves.[12] In the American context, many religiously based institutions in health care, education, and the social services focus their missions on special service to the poor and the otherwise marginalized. From this religious perspective, the vulnerabilities of poverty, sickness, and ignorance create a special spiritual opportunity, the potential for a link to the divine through service to the least well-off. Those providing care to these populations discharge a religious mission, one valued in itself.

This same point can be made in secular terms as well. It is a matter of moral common sense that fairness demands special advocacy for those least able to make their own voices heard. Wealthy, influential, and well-educated Americans will make their interests clear in any large social change, especially in debates about reform of the health care system. Middle class Americans, despite periodic feelings that "the system" is unresponsive to them, vote in large numbers and therefore have the attention of politicians who must seek re-election. Many of the least well-off, by contrast, are unsophisticated about politics and do not vote in large numbers. If their interests are to be defended effectively, others who are moved by a sense of fairness must champion their cause.

Social Justice

This simple insight of common-sense fairness can be made more formal through two different contemporary theories of social justice. Utilitarian theories hold that a just society is one that arranges its resources in such a way as to make the most people happy.[13] At the outset this may appear prejudicial against the interests of a minority, as securing the happiness of the majority would appear to be the easiest path to creating the greatest happiness for the greatest number. Often this is true. However, when wide disparities exist between the relative affluence and good health of the majority and the poverty and poor health of the minority, a surer route to increasing total happiness is to invest disproportionately in the needs of the least well-off. More dramatic gains are to be made there for less investment. It would take considerable investment, for example, to lower the infant morality rate substantially in an average affluent community where the rate is already low. Far fewer resources would be necessary to lower infant morality rates substantially in minority communities that have some of the highest rates of infant deaths.

This equalizing implication of utilitarianism can be clarified by a hypothetical scenario. Suppose a wealthy person inadvertently drops a twenty-dollar bill on the street. Later it is found by a person living near poverty. From one perspective, nothing of moment occurs in this situation except that twenty dollars passes from one person to another. From a utilitarian ethical perspective, however, the movement of the twenty dollars from a situation of plenty to one of need increases the power of the twenty dollars to buy happiness. On discovery of the loss of twenty dollars, the wealthy person might be confused and disappointed but, after all, he or she has more twenty-dollar bills to replace the one lost. On the other hand, the indigent person, on discovering the twenty-dollar bill, may be delighted by the prospect of being able to satisfy numerous unmet needs, including perhaps the basic needs of food, shelter, and clothing. The unhappiness experienced by the wealthy person is outweighed by the happiness experienced by the poor person. Therefore, moving resources from the wealthy to the poor can increase total happiness.

This utilitarian insight, that satisfying the needs of the least well-off can increase the overall happiness in society, also forms the general moral framework for progressive income taxation, citizens paying a higher percentage of their incomes in taxes as their incomes increase. Other things being equal and within certain limits, money that moves from the socioeconomic top of society to support the needs of those at the bottom can create more happiness than other tax schemes. Overall, the utilitarian theory of justice provides a reason to believe that a society is more just if it makes special efforts to ameliorate the conditions of those who are least well-off.

An Angelic Perspective

Another contemporary theory of justice provides support for the same conclusion, that efforts on behalf of the most vulnerable are morally imperative. This theory was set forth by American philosopher John Rawls.[14] It is a contemporary elaboration of the social contract theory developed by European thinkers in the Enlightenment period and articulated as early in the West as

Plato's *Crito*.[15] Rawls' version of the theory is complex, more complex than the present context requires or allows. Its central moral insight, however, can be conveyed easily by converting some of the main elements of Rawls' view into a creation myth.

Suppose an all-powerful creator God exists along with lesser spiritual beings or angels. (Although a strange supposition to a secular consciousness, this is an article of faith in many major world religions.) Angels can be conceived as intelligent, able to reason and choose.[16] Because they are wholly spiritual beings, however, they have no material existence; that is, they have no bodies. Consequently, they have none of the differences characteristic of embodied human beings, no differences in strength, physical beauty, age, or health. Suppose further that God's plan of creation involves placing each of these angels into a human body and putting them on earth to live together. In effect, the angels will become humans and experience all the diversity and inequalities associated with different degrees of strength, physical beauty, age, and health. Angels selected for this metamorphosis are told of their impending fate. They are also given a momentous opportunity. Before their embodiment, they are to meet to determine the outlines of justice for the society they are about to enter. God promises to enforce among the humans tomorrow whatever the angels agree to today.

Admittedly, these are fanciful assumptions, but an important moral point lies behind them. These assumptions allow for the creation of a hypothetical situation in which beings who can reason and choose, yet who have no specific knowledge of the inequalities they are about to experience, are given the task of determining the general elements of social justice. Put another way, this unusual set of circumstances allows for an examination of justice without the biases that are inevitable when real human beings debate issues of justice. It allows for a speculative exploration of moral reasoning freed from all preexisting prejudices.

How might angels in such a situation reason? Rawls argues that under a similar set of conditions (albeit without God and angels), rational beings would choose to make the lives they are about to lead the best those lives can be. They would do this by agreeing to maximize the minimal condition that fate, or in this scenario the will of God, may assign to any one of them. If this is so, each angel would therefore consider the worst possible condition that might be experienced under various possible social arrangements. Each angel would then refuse to agree to any arrangement unless the worst condition that arrangement produces is abolished altogether or improved to make it the "best worst" it can be. Each angel knows that the worst lot any angel gets could go to any angel and therefore wants even the worst condition to be the best it can be. For example, the angels would likely refuse to agree to racial slavery in their future reality on the grounds that, not knowing their future race, each could experience one of the worst conditions of slavery. Each would be motivated to avoid this fate by abolishing the institution of slavery altogether. If the society the angels agree to must have differences in wealth (perhaps to motivate effort and reward performance), they would want to make even the poorest condition the best it can be.

Consider how different the angels' reasoning might be if God allowed them knowledge of their race or wealth *before* the rules of justice are determined. It is just the ignorance of their specific differences (along with the general knowledge of what a difference these differences can make) that forces them to consider first the position of the least well-off person they can imagine. Each angel knows that he or she might be this worst-off person. Their strategy, then, is to abolish that worst position through mutual agreement or to seek ways to make that worst position the best it can be if for some good reasons it must exist. No doubt they would abolish racial slavery. If there were good reasons to allow differences in economic status, each would envision a future at the bottom of the economic ladder and strive mightily to make that condition the best it can be.

This creation myth is relevant in determining the outlines of justice in the health care system. If these angels were to consider the present health care system in the United States and were confronted with the possibility of being among the worst-off under it, they would seek to change the system dramatically. At the very least, they would try to soften the system's negative impact on the least well-off. No reasonable angel would accept a health care system in which he or she might be a member of a group that bears a disproportionate burden of society's morbidity and mortality and that must struggle with daunting problems of access, cost, and quality.

The moral point of this fanciful speculation should be clear. Nearly everyone wants to be fair. Yet we all see fairness through our own biases, including those shaped by socioeconomic status, racial and ethnic memberships, degree of education, condition of health, and so on. If all these inequalities could be stripped away, the question of fairness could be raised in its most elementary form: What would be fair to everyone if anyone could be subjected to the worst social conditions? Put this way, the demands of justice are clear because they are undistorted by bias.

This is precisely the perspective real people should try to assume because one of the rudimentary obligations of justice is to try to be as free of bias as possible.[17] Therefore, those seeking justice ought to take the perspective of the angels as a regulative ideal. In other words, when trying to determine the demands of social justice, considerations should begin with an assessment of the conditions of those who are least well-off. Each of us ought to ask whether we would regard society as fair if that worst condition were our own condition. If the answer is an emphatic no, then the work of justice must begin there.

At root, the perspective of the hypothetical angels provokes a Golden Rule insight.[18] Justice demands that social realities be assessed from the point of view of the other, especially from the other who is the least well-off. Applied to the context at hand, health care changes must be judged not simply by how they serve the interests of those who are already among the well-off and powerful in society, but by how they serve the interests of those who are the least well-off. Health care reform should aim for a system that makes the worst health care and health conditions the best they can be.

Barriers to Justice

There are serious inequities in the health care arena in the United States and strong religious and secular reasons for wanting to correct these inequities, for wanting to improve the situation of the least well-off. This conviction, however, is not persuasive to many Americans for several reasons. The most subterranean of these reasons is the persistence of racism and ethnic prejudice. Without putting it in so many words, perhaps even denying it were it made explicit, many Americans simply resist any efforts thought to be directed to the improvement of the lot of racial and ethnic minorities.[19] This view is obviously incompatible with the core of the Judeo–Christian tradition and the progressive ideals of the Enlightenment as well as with the specific theories of justice examined here. Nonetheless, racism is one of the abiding moral challenges in American life in general and in health care reform in particular. Little progress can be made in combatting it unless its influence is named, uncomfortable as that may be.

A second view, more respectable and therefore more frequently aired in contemporary political debates, although itself also deeply incompatible with the best in American religious and secular traditions, is a crude social Darwinism committed to a "dog-eat-dog" interpretation of society. This view is often rooted in a rugged individualism that denies the moral relevance of most social bonds.[20] Some versions recognize the significance of family and group connections but deny the relevance of moral obligations outside the immediacy of these intimate circles. This view is linked frequently with a heroic conception of success: Hard work inevitably brings success; poverty is the inevitable consequence of laziness and lack of self-discipline.[21] On this account, there is no justification for sympathy for the plight of the least well-off because those living in disadvantaged conditions deserve the circumstances in which they live. Their poverty is an expression of their own lack of effort. The poor need only exert the requisite will power and concerted effort to pull themselves out of their disadvantaged circumstances. Failure to do so is a continual moral indictment, not of society, but of the least well-off themselves.

A third cultural barrier to the conclusion that action on behalf of the least well-off is morally imperative is the most widespread. It may not be consistent with the dominant religious tradition, but it is consistent with some major themes in American secular traditions. In this view, the goal of greater equality for those living at the margins of society is admirable. The stark inequities in the United States should be softened or erased. The problem lies in appeal to government to achieve these goals. Whenever the government acts, it always entails unacceptable increases in taxation and regulation. Worse yet, government action to improve the worst conditions has proven itself to be ineffective, counterproductive, or both.[22]

In this view, the only acceptable weapons to combat the circumstances of the least well-off are voluntary efforts, education, and charity. Organized efforts on the part of government to provide services, to redistribute income, or to eradicate poverty have not succeeded and cannot do so. In the best cases, government efforts serve only to increase spending and swell bureaucracies. In the worst cases, the effect of government is to make its intended beneficiaries less self-reliant and therefore worse off than before government intervention. What is needed most is will power and self-reliance; what government creates is dependency.[23]

Removing Barriers

These are powerful barriers, but rejoinders can be made to each. Racial and ethnic prejudice is despicable and must be exposed for what it is. Although progress has not been nearly as rapid as justice demands, the United States has made important strides in this arena in the last several generations. The Civil Rights Movement ended racial barriers in the law and helped to make explicit public expressions of racism unacceptable culturally. The numbers of members of minority races and ethnic groups in positions of leadership and influence have grown throughout the United States. Genuine health care reform offers one of the few opportunities on the political horizon to make additional progress in this area in the near term. Creation of a system of universal access to high-quality health care for all Americans would be a clear and systemic rejection of racism. It would also be an important and symbolically powerful act of resistance to the slide toward "two Americas": an affluent, optimistic majority and an impoverished, alienated minority.[24]

With respect to the "dog-eat-dog" worldview, it is worth remembering the significant public subsidies that have supported the development and the delivery of health care since the end of World War II.[25] Substantial amounts of public money were spent on the expansion of the hospital sector and on efforts to increase the numbers of doctors. Massive subsidies from the tax system were used (and are still being used) to spread health insurance through the ranks of the middle classes. A great deal of money has been invested (and is still invested) in America's own federally run and tax-supported national health insurance program, Medicare. The rugged individualism assumed by the dog-eat-dog worldview is simply not applicable to health care. Furthermore, it is deeply incompatible with the basic orientation of caring that motivates the health care enterprise at its core. Health care is predicated on the dependence of people on one another. Nothing is more obvious in the face of serious or prolonged illness.

Finally, the lesson drawn by those who espouse the goal of improving the lot of the least well-off but reject the use of government as a means to that end, the lesson that government has shown itself inept, is simply overly broad. Certainly, some government programs have failed. Certainly, taxation and the spread of bureaucracy are substantive political issues that require debate and many prudential judgments; but the allegation that the federal government is simply incapable of creating a health care system that reduces or eliminates some of the most stark health status inequalities in the United States at an acceptable cost is belied by international experience. Nations around the world have accomplished this goal on their own terms.

No nation in the world is quite like the United States in every respect. Of course, this can be said equally about every other nation in the world. Nevertheless, many nations in the world share large portions of our national experience. Other nations have deep roots in the Judeo–Christian or the Enlightenment tradition or both. Others are immigrant nations or have marked racial and ethnic diversity. Others share our democratic politics and postindustrial economy. Others share our scientific–medical culture.

In virtually all the major trading partners of the United States who share some or all of these social realities, the government has erased the worst health care inequalities by creating universal health insurance coverage and by making special efforts on behalf of those who are least well-off in society. Not all of these international efforts succeed, nor are any of the successes transportable to the United States without adjustment for our American national experience and circumstances. Yet the fact remains that significant progress can be made in these areas because significant progress has been made elsewhere under reasonably similar conditions. Can health care reform be impossible for the United States, when it has been done with tolerable success by Canada, Japan, Germany, Great Britain, South Korea, Australia, France, Sweden, New Zealand, and others?

The view that the federal government is incompetent in the health care arena is also belied by domestic experience with the Medicare program. Since the mid-1960s, the United States has maintained a single national medical norm, a basic level of health care, for all elderly Americans regardless of medical conditions, socioeconomic circumstances, or state of residence. This achievement has strong political support, including the protection of the powerful American Association of Retired Persons (AARP). By and large, Americans regard Medicare as their own program, one that serves them and their families. There is little credible evidence that this age-linked national insurance program has created socially destructive dependencies or made people less concerned for their health because their care is insured. Certainly, there is room for greater efficiency and cost-consciousness in Medicare. Experiments with managed care, new forms of cost-sharing (especially for the wealthy elderly), and other cost-cutting measures are appropriate. There is no widespread public sentiment, however, to "get the government out" of Medicare, privatize it, or send it to the states. For all its flaws, the federal government has succeeded with Medicare, succeeded in creating and conducting a comprehensive national program of health coverage despite having focused on the most expensive phase of the life span.

Strategies for Justice

What exactly could the United States do to eliminate, or at least to mitigate, some of the worst health care conditions and to improve the lot of the least well-off Americans? Three general strategies suggest themselves. First, a universal health insurance system must be devised that includes a basic benefit package comprehensive enough to attract and maintain the support of the middle class so that the poor and the middle classes would rely on the same package. Even if some Americans who are very affluent would buy more coverage, the political power and influence of the middle class would assure that the basic benefit package is comprehensive and that the services covered by the benefit package are of high quality. In short, health care reform should tie the fate of the poor to that of the middle class.

Second, whatever health system evolves out of the present changes, greater investment must be made to address public health needs and to fund health initiatives in poorer communities. It would not be sufficient to achieve universal coverage without also responding to the fact that some areas of the nation and some groups would enter universal coverage with significant health status deficits and with significant insufficiencies in their health care delivery infrastructures.

Finally, to address these deficits, mechanisms would have to exist in a reformed health care system to draw health care professionals and resources toward underserved areas in both rural regions and the inner cities, perhaps by creating enhanced reimbursements for providers in those areas. Efforts like the National Health Service Core, which provides scholarships to medical students in exchange for future service in underserved areas, could be expanded.[26] Financial arrangements are needed to underwrite the ability of institutions in these communities to purchase needed medical equipment and to upgrade physical plants. This is especially imperative for academic health centers, which provide a great deal of uncompensated care in America's largest cities. Because of this financial drain and the costs of their educational programs, academic health centers are unwelcome partners in emerging health care networks. They are therefore at a significant disadvantage in a competitive environment.[27] As a general strategy, more must be done to support institutions and professionals who serve the underserved. Commitment to improving the lot of the least well-off means adopting affirmative action measures within a general commitment to the human equality dictated by respect for human dignity.

It is obvious that present changes in the health care marketplace will not and cannot achieve these goals. Competition and cost-cutting will not bring universal coverage or health care affirmative action. In fact, they are very likely to make the situation worse. Markets alone cannot serve the interests of the least well-off. Despite American reluctance to admit the point, the logic of markets, worldwide health care experience, and the success of Medicare indicate both the necessity and possibility of government action in this arena.

The Sick and Dying

There is one additional category of vulnerable Americans whose plight deserves special emphasis as the health care system evolves. Ironically, these are the sick and the dying, Americans who have been the traditional focus of the health care system. This could change, and to their disadvantage. In the present climate, it is not uncommon for critics from all political leanings to condemn the entire health care system as a "sick care system."[28] These critics demand greater emphasis on prevention and wellness programs. Certainly, they have a point. Prevention and wellness are indeed understressed in the present system, and more should be done in this arena. Yet it is worth remembering that the primary clients for prevention and wellness programs are healthy people, those who are already well-off in health care terms.

At the same time, one of the most important and growing influences in the new health care marketplace is capitation. The main financial incentive at the heart of capitation provides a very strong temptation to enroll healthy, underutilizing populations and to avoid or disenroll sick, overutilizing populations. Healthy people pay their monthly fees and make no claims on the capitated network's resources. The sick and dying, by contrast, are loss leaders from a financial perspective; they drain resources from the network.

Greater stress on prevention and the financial incentives of capitation therefore threaten the traditional commitment of the system to the care of those
most in need, the sick and the dying.

There is much to be said in favor of both prevention and capitation. It is
certainly true that American health care could do far more to prevent illness
and to keep Americans well. All things considered, it is better to prevent illness than to perfect means of dealing with it when it occurs, but not all illness is preventable in every case, and dying is not preventable in any case.
Regardless of preventive efforts, there will always be sick and dying patients
in need of assistance from the health care system. In the rush to develop more
wellness programs and to keep people out of hospitals, this important fact
must not be forgotten. Regrettable though it may be, most people are not
interested in health and health care when they are healthy. It is when they
are sick, and especially when they are dying, that people need health care
and the services of dedicated professionals and institutions.

There are many benefits to be expected from capitation, not the least of
which is the incentive in networks to keep enrollees healthy, an incentive
suggested by the term "health maintenance organization." Efforts today to keep
enrollees free of disease tomorrow can serve the financial interests of a
capitated plan. Capitation can also be expected to increase economic efficiency. Care for the most vulnerable, however, means that capitated networks
must be carefully regulated to avoid abuses: disenrollment of those who need
them most, use of preexisting illness exclusions, and adoption of marketing
techniques that are designed to build a network profile of healthy underutilizing enrollees. Ways will have to be developed to curb these abuses, from
simple legal prohibition of disenrollment and preexisting illness exclusions
to risk-adjusted reimbursement and incentives or mandates to enroll high-risk
populations.

In the years ahead there will be considerable experimentation with preventive programs and ways to control the negative side of capitation. Throughout this experimentation, the moral goal must be clear. A special value and a
special obligation are associated with care of the most vulnerable, the least
well-off. In health care, the primary focus must remain on care of the sick and
the dying. They have a special right to health care, and society has a special
duty to care for them.

Notes

1. Robert E. Goodin, *Protecting the Vulnerable* (Chicago: University of Chicago
   Press, 1985), 6–8.
2. Goodin, *Protecting the Vulnerable*, pp. 110–17.

3. See, generally, Charles J. Dougherty and Sandra L. Dougherty, "Moral Reconstruction in the Hospital: A Legal and Philosophical Perspective on Patient Rights," *Creighton Law Review* 14, no. 4, supplement (1980-1981): 1409-1434.

4. Dougherty, "Equality and Inequality in American Health Care," pp. 6-17; and Lu Ann Aday, *At Risk in America* (San Francisco: Jossey-Bass, 1993).

5. Dougherty, *American Health Care*, pp. 3-19.

6. Ibid., p. 5.

7. *A Matter of Fact* 19 (July-December 1993) (Ann Arbor, Mich.: Pierian Press, 1994), 108-109.

8. J. Morris, D. Cook, and A. Shaper, "Loss of Employment and Mortality," *British Medical Journal* 308, no. 6937 (1994): 1135-39; D. Ezzy, "Unemployment and Mental Health: A Critical Review," *Social Science and Medicine* 37, no. 1 (1993): 41-52; and S. Wilson and G. Walker, "Unemployment and Health: A Review," *Public Health* 107, no. 3 (1993): 153-62.

9. *A Matter of Fact,* 17 (July-December 1992) (Ann Arbor, Mich.: Pierian Press, 1993), 188.

10. Daniel Callahan, "Reforming the Health Care System for Children and the Elderly to Balance Cure and Care," *Academic Medicine* 67, no. 4 (1992): 219-22.

11. Generally, see Robert Murray, *The Cosmic Covenant: Biblical Themes of Justice, Peace, and the Integrity of Creation* (London: Sheed and Ward, 1992).

12. Paul Maier, *First Christians: Pentecost and the Spread of Christianity* (New York: Harper and Row, 1976).

13. The classic source is John Stuart Mill, *Utilitarianism*, ed. Samuel Gorovitz (Indianapolis: Bobbs-Merrill, 1971).

14. John Rawls, *A Theory of Justice* (Cambridge, Mass.: Harvard University Press, 1971); H. Gene Blocker and Elizabeth H. Smith, *John Rawls' Theory of Justice* (Athens, Ohio: Ohio University Press, 1980).

15. For a treatment of the social contract thinkers in Enlightenment, see Michael Lessnoff, *Social Contract* (Atlantic Highlands, N.J.: Humanities Press International, 1986). *Crito* is in Plato, *The Collected Dialogues*, ed. E. Hamilton and H. Cairns (Princeton, N.J.: Princeton University Press, 1961), 27-39.

16. See, e.g., James Collins, *The Thomistic Philosophy of Angels* (Washington, D.C.: Catholic University Press, 1947).

17. Louis Katzner, "The Original Position and the Veil of Ignorance," in Blocker and Smith, eds. *John Rawls' Theory of Justice*, pp. 42-70.

18. See, e.g., Sissela Bok, *Lying* (New York: Vintage Books, 1979), 30-32.

19. See, e.g., Joseph A. Califano, "The Challenge to the Health Care System: Can the Third Biggest Business Take Care of the Medically Indigent? A Personal Perspective," in *Health Care for the Poor and Elderly: Meeting the Challenge*, ed. Duncan Yaggy (Durham, N.C.: Duke University Press, 1984), 45-57.

20. Dougherty, "The Excesses of Individualism," pp. 22-28.

21. Majorie Hope and James Young, *The Faces of Homelessness* (Lexington, Mass.: Lexington Books), pp. 197-201.

22. On expanding government bureaucracies, see Robert Higgs, *Crisis and Leviathan: Critical Episodes in the Growth of American Government* (New York: Oxford University Press, 1987); and James Q. Wilson, *Bureaucracy: What Government Agencies Do and Why They Do It* (New York: Basic Books, 1989).

23. On the problem of dependency, see June Axinn and Mark Stern, *Dependency and Poverty: Old Problems in a New World* (Lexington, Massachusetts: Lex-

ington Books, 1988); and Tamar Ann Mehuron, editor, *Points of Light: New Approaches to Ending Welfare Dependency* (Washington, D.C.: Ethics and Public Policy Center, 1991).

24. Fred R. Harris and Roger W. Wilkins, eds., *Quiet Riots: Race and Poverty in the United States* (New York: Pantheon Books, 1988); and Bill E. Lawson, *The Underclass Question* (Philadelphia: Temple University Press, 1992).

25. Starr, *Social Transformation of American Medicine*, pp. 335-378.

26. V. Stone, J. Brown, and V. Sidel, "Decreasing the Field Strength of the National Health Service Corps: Will Access to Care Suffer?" *Journal of Health Care for the Poor and Underserved* 2, no. 3 (1991): 347-58.

27. J. Jonas, S. Etzel, and B. Barzansky, "Educational Programs in US Medical Schools, 1993-1994," *JAMA* 272, no. 9 (1994): 694-701; and John K. Iglehart, "Health Care Reform and Graduate Medical Education," *The New England Journal of Medicine* 330, no. 16 (1994): 1167-71.

28. See, e.g., E. Bevis, "Alliance for Destiny: Education and Practice," *Nursing Management* 24, no. 4 (1993): 56-61.

6

The Common Good

Individualism

Commitment to the value of human dignity supports the obligation to respect each individual person. This is not only an American cultural disposition, but also has the force of law. It has become such a prominent feature in our national experience in the second half of the twentieth century that it is accurate, if ironic, to observe that American society is highly individualistic.[1]

American legal commitment to rights frequently entails the vindication of individuals' rights against the interests of groups. Public policy options are often shaped and limited by concern about their potential impact on individuals. Protection of individual privacy and deference to self-determination have created a wide range of personal freedoms, particularly in lifestyle and sexuality, and have profoundly altered many traditional relationships. These changes have been positive in many ways. Their link to the value of human dignity is a legitimate source of pride for the entire nation.

However, there is a negative side. As the century draws to a close, there is a palpable sense of fragmentation and rootlessness in American life. Major institutions—the family, churches, voluntary associations—are under unprecedented stress.[2] Despite considerable progress in some areas, racial and class differences have been exacerbated in other areas and have become fertile ground for a harvest of hopelessness and violence.[3] The considerable strides women have made in removing unjust gender barriers to achievement and in bringing new sensitivities to the working environment have been followed in many cases by new forms of gender distrust and bitterness.[4] Affirmative action programs that have benefitted many women and members of minorities are increasingly met with resentment by white males and attacked as reverse discrimination. Many of the most fundamental relationships in society—in the family, in schools, in health care—have been entangled with litigation and fears of legal liability.[5] There is a growing sense that the achievements of individualism have been financed by the loss of social context and community.

Persons and Society

This need not be the case. Respect for dignity does not require commitment to excessive individualism, although it plainly demands respect for individual persons. Instead, an adequate appreciation of the value of dignity must do justice to the full nature of persons, including social dimensions. Individuals are shaped in societies, especially by the family, school, and workplace. Success or failure of these societies and the relationships and institutions that compose them sets the stage for the satisfaction or frustration of individuals. The ability to become an individual in any meaningful sense requires successful socialization.[6] Development of a person with interior depth of thought and feeling and with the ability to be self-determining is a collective achievement, requiring successes in many societies. A culture that ignores this social context and glorifies the lone individual not only misses these evident realities, but also undermines the concrete processes needed to build and maintain individuals.

Those concrete social processes begin with biology, where it is literally true that the individual is heir to the collective success of the species. This point is graphic in the metaphor of a gene pool. The first important social relationship of life is that between a fetus and the woman who carries him or her.[7] Much is determined about the future prospects of individuals by the character of this relationship, which is itself shaped in important ways by the general social conditions facing the pregnant woman. Overall state of health, age, and access to prenatal care are obviously critical, but these factors are themselves often affected by relationships with family and friends and by the socioeconomic and cultural conditions that supply or threaten physical and emotional security.

The quality of relationships that support the growing child after birth and through a long period of dependence is deeply important. Emotional life is structured and personality formed in daily encounters with others. The self is shaped most intimately by the acquisition of language in childhood because in the development of this skill an individual gains access to external and internal worlds simultaneously. The beginning of the ability to speak with others, to understand and convey meanings to others, is at the same time the dawn of the ability to form internal speech, which means entering a form of life and beginning to build a self.[8] The character of the institutional structure that surrounds this early learning, namely, the family, schools, and neighborhood, make a great deal of difference in a person's destiny. Without denying the important phenomena of individual choice and personal responsibility, these early factors in the social environment help to determine the direction of an individual's life. Consider, for example, the difference in life prospects between a child born to an affluent, professional family in an American suburb and a child born to a single mother on welfare in the inner city. It is not impossible, of course, for the first child to fail despite these advantages and for the second child to succeed despite these disadvantages; but the odds are plainly stacked against this occurrence in both cases.

The social stamp of early development continues in more subtle ways throughout an individual's life. Loves, friendships, working relationships, and the institutional patterns that support and shape particular relationships all continue to make, and in some cases unmake, persons throughout their adult lives. That such obvious facts deserve mention at this time in American national life is a tribute to the stress now placed on the image of the individual autonomously choosing a specific path in the world; but individualism, autonomy, and even informed consent are all deeply rooted in social life.

Foundations

One value closely linked to the social nature of persons is commitment to the common good, a concern for and service to a community larger than the individual and that individual's immediate groupings. Traditionally, the value of the common good has had a strong appeal. Loyalties as diverse as teamwork on the job, patriotism, and environmental activism all embody a core value of service to the common good. The challenge for Americans is to make sense of this traditional value in a plural and individualistic culture.[9] What is the meaning of *the* common good in a society of many cultures, especially at a time when diversity is not viewed as a challenge to be overcome (the "melting pot") but a fact to be celebrated? Certainly, individuals have their private goods and families and circles of friends, their quasiprivate goods. The goods pertaining to racial, ethnic, and gender memberships, to region, corporation, church, professional or civic associations are common; yet these are not the common good of a whole society. In fact, pursuit of these goods is often consciously in opposition to others' interpretation of society's common good.

Worse yet, the individualism and consequent value relativism that dominate American society make discussion of the common good not merely difficult but often offensive. To many, the notion of the common good portends the imposition of someone else's values, conformism, even authoritarianism. It evokes a defensive "who are you to say what's good for me" response. The objection is not so much that someone pursuing the common good may get it wrong, may misinterpret the true common good. Competing interpretations of the common good is an issue for all societies. The special challenge to contemporary Americans is the very possibility of a common good, as if national life were predicated on foreswearing discussion of any goods beyond those pursued by individuals. Yet there must be moments when the question of what is good for *us* can and must be asked. The size, character, and stakes of the health care system make it a natural focus for this question.

There is an important lesson, however, in American caution about the notion of the common good. Whatever content is given to the notion must be provisional, historical, self-consciously open to future development.[10] It must be vague and therefore subject to containing simultaneously elements that are in tension with one other, perhaps some that are contradictory. Yet it must also provide a sense of general direction for society, targets or benchmarks for progress. Substantively, conceptions of the common good and service driven by them will be shaped by the particulars of various arenas of life and the projects associated with them, for example, a specific task at work, a public policy challenge for the nation, the details of a plan to protect the environment. Little can be said generally about the content of the common good separate from these many contexts. However, three structural elements of the common good shape any recognizable meaning of the notion.[11]

The common good must acknowledge or create a community of persons. It must, that is, be based on something real held in common. The common good is rooted in membership and therefore contains a rudimentary presumption of equality. Obviously, people can be members of groups in different ways; community does not entail sameness. In the contemporary world, however, acknowledgment of a community of persons must be based on the equal moral membership entailed by the value of human dignity: Each person has incalculable worth. A nation could not serve its own common good by ignoring or persecuting persons in its own national community. (This point sheds some light on the tendency to deny the personhood of those who are ignored or persecuted in the context of a distorted notion of the common good.)

The common good must prize freedom. One of the most distinctive goods a society can provide is deference to a wide range of freedom. This is a hard-won lesson in human history, especially in this century. Freedom is not the only good that life in common provides; many others are richer and deeper by far. Nonetheless, few other goods retain their goodness when freedom is not prized. Freedom in this context means, in the first place, personal liberty and the basic human rights associated with it, but it also means the cultivation of multiple autonomous associations in society, the flourishing of a pluralism of production, creativity, and power.

Finally, the common good must generate and share mutual benefits that can be shared. There must be a net gain to all from life together, and that gain must be distributed equitably. When social sacrifices are required, they must be shared equitably as well. This most substantive aspect of the common good must include many and varying goods that cannot be named in advance of real situations. Nevertheless, mutual benefits in contemporary industrial democracies must include fair sharing of both material and spiritual goods. The former includes the basic securities demanded by human vulnerability: food, clothing, shelter, education, employment, and health care. The latter includes the refinements made possible by the human drive for excellence, such as art, science, culture, personal growth, and entertainment. The meaning of equity in the distribution of these goods is itself a vexing question. Some direction is suggested, however, by the links of the value of the common good to caring (about the community) and to concern for the least well-off (as persons). A society in which some persons share little in some or all or these categories would have a flawed or impoverished sense of its own common good as a community.

Health and Health Care

Application of the value of the common good in health care begins with an understanding of how much of health care is a common good, a social achievement. Despite the fact that individuals can make a difference in their own health and the health of their families and communities, it is plain that a great deal of the positive improvement in health status in the twentieth century in industrialized nations has come from access to clean water, improved sewer systems, and enhanced nutrition.[12] These changes represent collective achievements of communities, not simply individual efforts. Public health measures to control infections have also been remarkably successful, securing collective protections against diseases that are very difficult to combat with personal initiative alone.

Even acts of health promotion that are under the immediate control of individuals—choices about smoking, drinking, eating, and exercise, for example—have important social dimensions.[13] Patterns of drinking and eating, for example, have obvious ethnic links. Patterns of cigarette smoking demonstrate socioeconomic, regional, gender, and age dimensions. Appreciation of the importance of exercise is plainly a result of multiple health promotion efforts. Knowledge about and access to healthy foods, especially fruits and vegetables, also reveal cultural differences.

Similar points about the importance of social context can be made about the providers' side of health care. Doctors, nurses, and other health care professionals sacrifice a great deal for their degrees and are typically hardworking, dedicated individuals. Given these realities, it is easy to forget the social context that makes their individual efforts possible. Health care is built on generations of scientific efforts in basic research, experimentation with animals and human subjects, collection and analysis of data, theory formation, and educational efforts.

Compared with most other human endeavors, the health sciences have displayed an exceptional degree of altruism and concern for the common good. There have been marked intrusions of business practices into the health sciences, for example, the guarding of proprietary information, controlling pharmaceutical and medical devices with patents, and withholding potentially important breakthroughs from professional colleagues for pecuniary gain.[14] Nevertheless, this behavior is more the exception than the rule in the histories of the health sciences and health care. In contrast to the general patterns of conduct in the business world, health care practitioners and scientists in related areas have freely shared important breakthroughs with others and have taken steps to make beneficial products and services widely available to other health care providers and the public. The very fact that so much has been written in the last generation about the surprising rise of frank entrepreneurial activity within the health sciences (especially in biology and genetics) is itself a testament to how relatively rare such behavior has been in the past.[15] As a rule, knowledge relevant to the prevention of disease, the preservation of life, and the amelioration of human suffering has been thought to have a collective rather than a private character. Regardless of their hard work and dedication, today's doctors, nurses, pharmacists would have little power to benefit their patients were it not for this common intellectual inheritance.

The provider infrastructure is itself the result of considerable public efforts. Although new forces are changing this institution, for most of the second half of the twentieth century, hospitals have been doctors' workshops. Many of these impressive institutions were built or expanded after World War II with federal funds made available by the Hill–Burton Act.[16] At the same time, the federal government invested heavily in American medical schools with the goal of increasing the supply of doctors. Federal policy was also important in attracting many doctors educated at foreign medical schools to practice in the United States; they now constitute one of every four practicing doctors in the nation.[17]

Public dollars were also very important in the financing of health care in the second part of the twentieth century. After World War II, the U.S. government used generous tax subsidies to provide an incentive for the spread of private health insurance linked to employment.[18] In the mid–1960s, the introduction of Medicare and Medicaid introduced large-scale public funding into the system to provide for the care of the elderly (Medicare) and the poor (Medicaid). The Medicare program was particularly generous, paying "usual, customary, and reasonable" rates and imposing few restrictions on reimbursement until the prospective payment or DRG system in the mid-1980s.[19] Moreover, despite the widespread impression that Medicare enrollees are only getting back money they have paid into the program during their working years, Medicare is heavily subsidized with public funds. Contributions made to the program by current enrollees cover less than a third of the projected costs of their lifetime benefits.[20] Public policy was also instrumental in the more recent spread of HMOs and other systems of capitation and managed care.[21] The U.S. government has also invested billions in biomedical research, generating medical advances and creating a massive new industry.

This social context is transparent and thus too often overlooked. After applying considerable skill throughout a long and difficult procedure, a surgeon may believe that the central contribution in assuring a good outcome for the patient is on the part of the surgeon. A nurse in the recovery room may regard the nursing effort as the most critically important part of the patient's postoperative care. The hospital administrator may feel a special personal pride in effectively managing the resources of a large institution in support of the surgeon, nurse, and patient. The insurance reviewer monitoring reimbursement for the procedure may take credit for maintaining fiscal discipline while honoring contractual commitments. The patient may feel that his or her personal efforts and healthy habits set the stage for a successful outcome and return to health. All these perspectives may be true in part, but they are surely incomplete. Each perspective lacks an awareness of the social dimension of each activity and the public investment that makes success in these endeavors possible.

Utilitarianism

How is this social dimension of health care best elaborated and evaluated from a moral perspective? How is the common good best understood in the health care arena? One obvious and direct approach to these issues is available by use of the utilitarian ethical framework. It has already been shown how utilitarian reasoning can provide theoretical support for improving the circumstances of the least well-off in society; such a strategy can increase net happiness. Utilitarianism is also a natural interpretative framework for the common good because it is based on aggregate reasoning (the *common* good) and focused on producing maximal benefit (the common *good*).

According to the utilitarian theory, all moral obligation is determined by reference to the projected consequences of alternative courses of action for all those affected by the acts under consideration.[22] To act morally in any given situation, an agent is duty bound to identify alternative courses of action, including none at all, and to trace out imaginatively the likely impact of each alternative. The morally responsible agent then must choose the one course of action that appears to provide the optimal set of outcomes, where "optimal" means producing the most benefit, the least harm, or, as in most cases, the best ratio of benefit to harm for all those affected by the choice. Among the chief virtues of utilitarianism is its responsiveness to context. Moral absolutes are rejected in favor of assessment of the situation and its possible futures.

Utilitarianism does not exclude consideration of the interests of the agent, but counts that interest as one of many, allowing for the obvious fact that the intensity of various consequences on those affected may vary considerably and in many cases will be very strongly centered directly on the agent. Nevertheless, the utilitarian understanding of moral obligation is inherently other-directed inasmuch as the focus is on outcome and a rational assessment of aggregate benefits and harms for all those involved. Thus, utilitarianism is committed to "the greatest good for the greatest number." This is a formula that appears to put utilitarianism squarely in the service of the common good. Utilitarianism would also provide a relatively clear standard for health care reform: to create whatever pattern of access to services creates the most happiness.

It is probably fair to say that no genuine commitment to the common good can do without a utilitarian element. Assessment of what is in the best interest of a society at any given time must involve strategies akin to utilitarian analysis. Nevertheless, there are at least three reasons why the common good is not best understood and promoted in an exclusively utilitarian fashion.[23]

Limits of Utility

First, there is a rather practical objection to utilitarian reasoning. For any but the most deliberate of choices, the kind of speculative and comprehensive reasoning required by a utilitarian analysis simply is not possible. Most moral action requires a certain degree of decisiveness. Choices must be made in a given window of opportunity. Rare are the occasions when alternatives can be carefully laid out and their consequences articulated and weighed one against another. Choices about marriage and careers are sometimes made in this fashion, but clearly they are exceptional cases. Even in these cases, projections into the future are cloudy at best. Moreover, in contrast to the high degree of rational reflection that utilitarianism requires, most ethical choices rely to a great extent on feelings, habits, and intuitions or hunches.

In some versions of utilitarianism, these practical problems are addressed by composing a set of moral rules that are themselves justified periodically by reference to the principle of utility. Agents then follow these rules without utilitarian assessment in the context of choice, with confidence that overall and in the long run the application of these moral rules in varying circumstances will serve the greatest good for the greatest number. This strategy, referred to as rule utilitarianism, certainly does help to address the practical objections. It simplifies ethical decision-making and therefore does greater justice to the exigencies of choice; but rule utilitarianism becomes problematic in situations in which moral rules conflict with one another, one of the most frequent problems in moral experience. The rule utilitarian must then appeal directly to the principle of utility, tracing out the consequences of the use of alternative rules to determine which creates the greatest good for the greatest number in this case; but this recreates the practical problems at hand. Furthermore, the very flexibility and responsiveness to context that are the chief virtues of utilitarianism are threatened or lost by commitment to a set of moral rules, even if the rules themselves are subject to periodic utilitarian inspection. In the context of choice, the rules are definitive. A serious rule utilitarian can be just as inflexible as the most hidebound traditionalist.

Utilitarianism also has a problem in the articulation of benefits and harms to others, the empirical bedrock of the theory. If benefits and harms are understood in a straightforward descriptive sense—how people most likely will react to what they experience—then utilitarianism may lead to some very unorthodox conclusions. A utilitarian, for example, might hesitate to offend the attitudes of individuals known to be racists because moral criticism would create unhappiness. In fact, any moral judgment about any action could be made only on utilitarian grounds, that is, on the presumption that the judgment itself would do more good than harm. Furthermore, utilitarians can, indeed must, violate all the ordinary moral rules when the consequences demand it. Murder, theft, rape, lying, and similar acts could be morally permissible, even mandatory, if they appear to be the means of attaining the best outcome possible in a situation. For ordinary people of good moral sense, this implication of the theory turns the virtue of flexibility into a vice.

On the other hand, if benefits and harms are not straightforward but are assumed to be malleable over time, then utilitarianism has truly unpredictable implications. Suppose, for example, that in the future people could feel happy or neutral about things that today make people profoundly unhappy. This would make benefit and harm far too subjective and relative a basis on which to base assessment of the common good. Consider an extreme example. The conduct of Adolph Hitler toward the Jews is widely condemned on moral grounds. That his program of genocide was wrong, in fact, a moral abomination, is one of the most secure moral judgments of this age. Utilitarians can account for this consensus by pointing to the great suffering this policy caused. Suppose, however, that Hitler had won the Second World War and had succeeded in his plan to destroy European Jewry. In time, there would be a dwindling memory of the community he had destroyed and the millions of lives he had taken. Perhaps evidence of this atrocity would have been destroyed and lost to historical record. Generations born after the war would be taught that the genocide had been a necessity; given the character of Nazi propaganda, this monumental evil would even be presented as heroic. Under these (admittedly counterfactual) assumptions, fewer people would feel pain at the idea of Nazi genocide and more would take pleasure in it. Would a utilitarian analysis then have to conclude that genocide had become morally right?

A similar paradox can be generated without fanciful speculations simply by starting from the real history of the post-World War II period. Each year there are deaths in the group of those most immediately affected by the Holocaust, namely, survivors and their loved ones. Each year, therefore, brings less concrete memory of the sufferings this brutality caused. Must utilitarians hold that the Holocaust of European Jews becomes less wrong each year as fewer people are alive who suffered directly from it?

These possibilities suggest that utilitarianism fails to capture an immediate and natural moral intuition that even when its harms are past and even if latter generations were to perceive only benefits from it, genocide is something wrong in itself, a moral abomination. Utilitarian appeal to happiness and unhappiness as the final and exclusive arbiters of right and wrong therefore commits it to variety of relativism that seems intolerable in the face of a massive evil, the wrongfulness of which is one of the most deeply held moral convictions of modern times.

The final inadequacy of utilitarianism is that its form of emphasis on the common good may undermine the first value identified here: respect for human dignity. There is a potential in any utilitarian analysis for what John Stuart Mill called the "tyranny of the majority."[24] It would be hard, for example, to envision a society committed thoroughly to utilitarian principles that would be able or willing at the same time to articulate and guarantee a set of individual rights. A person can have a right on utilitarian grounds only to the extent that it produces the greatest good for all. This is a fragile basis for rights and distant from the standard view that rights are entitlements that persons have regardless of the consequences for others.[25] Again, there is the possibility of adopting a rule utilitarian approach that might regard individual rights as social rules that are better not violated for the sake of long-term utility. Nevertheless, when the (apparent) overall and long-term consequences for the majority dictate it, these rules themselves are subject to change. Even the rule utilitarian approach, therefore, seems not to capture the primary reason why human rights are important, namely, because they protect the inherent dignity of each person whether or not such protection maximizes the greatest good for the greatest number. The common good cannot be served by a view that relies so heavily on reasoning about aggregate interests.

Correcting Utilitarianism

Although it may sound ironic, the common good can be served only by a central commitment to respect the dignity of individual persons.[26] The three difficulties with utilitarianism can be addressed by moderating utilitarian analysis with an independent commitment to respect individual rights. Plainly, the addition of individual rights addresses the problem of the tyranny of the majority, as these rights limit the scope of majoritarian rule. Fundamental rights cannot be violated even if such violations appear to promote the greatest good. There may indeed be truly catastrophic circumstances when protection of society against serious and imminent harms can justify the temporary suspension of rights. Abraham Lincoln's suspension of habeas corpus, an action that in effect violated the right to be free from arbitrary arrest and confinement, is a case in point.[27] This extreme step was justified by an extreme set of circumstances: the perils of civil war. Admitting the possibility of an exception to avoid tragedy is a different matter from grounding the entire structure of individual rights on the consequences they have for everyone. The only proper and secure foundation for rights is the dignity of each person.

When there is a structure of individual rights that must be respected prior to attempts to maximize happiness, problems associated with the relativity of benefit and harm are resolved as well. Some acts are wrong regardless of what others think or feel about them, simply because they are disrespectful of persons; murder and genocide are obvious examples. Finally, some of the practical problems related to decision-making are also resolved because not every moral choice requires the rigors of a utilitarian analysis. Theft and lying are wrong because they undermine respect for persons. No lengthy analysis of consequences is needed to make this point. Again, difficult situations may arise that call for exceptions: a theft of documents to help a nation defend itself against potential aggression, a lie that saves a life. Even in these cases, however, moral analysis must begin not with appeal to consequences, but with the presumption that such acts are generally wrong in themselves.

From a theoretical perspective, utilitarianism and respect for individual rights are incompatible insights: One is primarily social, whereas the other stresses the individual. Yet both insights are needed from a practical point of view. Commitment to human dignity without a vision of the good of the whole, a vision characteristic of utilitarianism, yields only an extreme individualism detached from the realities that create and shape real persons. Exclusive emphasis on utilitarianism, by contrast, provides support for the common good in a statistical sense. Yet it fails to do justice to the one aspect of the common good that is nonnegotiable at the start of the twenty-first century, namely, that the good of society as a whole is linked to its respect for each individual person. This is one of the main lessons to be drawn from the twentieth century's catastrophic experimentation with totalitarianisms of the right and left.[28]

What is needed is a simultaneous commitment to perspectives that are by their nature in tension with each other, a commitment to persons and to society. Some may dismiss this as contradictory. Yet living and struggling with "contradictions" of this sort seem to be part of the traditional wisdom that holds that success lies in striking a creative balance between opposing insights. Personal freedom, for example, requires discipline or else it dissolves into license. Successful parenting must be both challenging and supportive. Corporate success demands simultaneous attention to process and to the product or service produced. Significant artistic achievement captures both order and chaos. Success at most tasks requires both attention to detail and a sense of the whole. Life itself dictates perseverance and rest, work and play. Thus, although it may seem from a strictly theoretical point of view to be inconsistent to hold both a social utilitarian insight and a commitment to the dignity of individual persons, this dual view is the expression in political philosophy of a familiar demand of practical wisdom.

Balance

This position is essentially Aristotelian: Moral virtue and all types of excellence are achieved by balancing and negotiating between extremes.[29] Imbalances must be diagnosed and new balances struck by "leaning against" the extreme that is overstressed. If this is true, if "the golden mean" of virtue requires setting a balance between opposing tendencies, then an ethical prescription for charting the common good of society must be situated in the context at hand. It must be sensitive to the problem, the place, and the time.

Understanding the details of the problem at hand is significant because this is what gives rise to ethical inquiry and delimits the range of possible solutions. For example, finding the right balance in a situation where conflict exists between individual rights and the good of society must begin with attention to the nature of the imbalance at hand. Perhaps there is a sense that a right has been violated or that a claim of right has been expanded beyond its historical or natural scope. The way the problem is understood and articulated makes some strategies for improvement more immediately viable and others less so. Place is clearly relevant, as different communities, especially ethnic and national communities, have inherited a given balance between concern for society and respect for the individual and are therefore subject to particular kinds of challenges to that inherited balance. Finally, time is critical because a community's and a person's sense of balance even on the most basic of issues is subject to evolution over time. For example, the balance between society and individual set in the United States of the 1790s is continuous with, yet dramatically different from, the same balance struck in the 1890s and 1990s.

Application of this stereoscopic vision must therefore begin with an honest assessment of existing imbalances. As argued above, there are many reasons to believe that the current imbalance facing the United States is a tilt too far in the direction of the individual and away from concerns for the common good. Therefore, resolution of many difficult moral problems will require a leaning against the individual toward what serves the interest of communities, what promotes the greatest good for the greatest number. This must be a practical disposition, not a total theoretical commitment to utilitarianism because there must remain a vital commitment to the dignity of each individual person.

Informed consent provides a useful example. Its emergence and domination represent a clear triumph of the value of the patient's individual dignity in the doctor–patient relationship. This is a distinctive contribution of American culture and one that should be protected. Yet there are many signs that the notion of informed consent has become artificial and in some cases destructive of trust in the doctor–patient relationship.[30] Many younger doctors who were educated in the world of patient autonomy appear to believe that their primary professional responsibility is only to provide information and to perform the services desired by the patient. They seem uncomfortable with giving advice, especially about urging their own opinions about the best course of treatment for their patients. To do so seems to them incompatible with the spirit of informed consent, that is, that the patient must give free and informed consent.[31]

In this climate of opinion, the shared and contextual character of decision-making must be stressed to balance an abstract notion of patient indepen-

dence. Patients rely on their doctors for professional advice. Some must be
persuaded to take the course that is medically best for them. This is especially
clear in rehabilitation.[32] Many young adults who have been through a paralyzing trauma reject proposed rehabilitation; in such circumstances, it is often
clear to the physiatrist and family that rehabilitation is in the patient's best
interest. When this is so, it would be morally irresponsible simply to defer to
the informed rejection of the patient. In such cases, "active persuasion" can
be justified. This is a social reality about patients, families, and doctors. Providing the kind of practical help patients need in making decisions can be
accomplished without violating their right to informed consent, but only if a
more socially realistic view of informed consent is assumed.

If this general assessment is correct, namely, that a tilt in favor of society is
appropriate because of the current overemphasis on the individual, then this
disposition should become a guiding principle in contemporary medical ethics. Two important provisos must be added to this conclusion. First, sensitivity to context will demand that this guiding assumption be dropped in some
cases where the rights of individuals continue to need vindication and too
much emphasis has already been placed on society. Furthermore, an assessment of this sort is one that must be redone periodically because a society
that overstresses the individual at one time may incline in the opposite direction at another time.

Second, people of goodwill can differ not only on the general assessment
of the imbalance facing our society, but also on the matter of degree of the
imbalance. How much of an imbalance favoring the individual exists now in
the United States, and therefore how much attention to society is needed to
retrieve balance? Moreover, specific moral problems can be so complex and
require so much practical judgment that even those who share the same social diagnosis may disagree on its application to the case at hand. In spite of
these qualifications, the point remains that in the United States in general and
in health care in particular, an excessive individualism now prevails. The cure
for this malady is to give greater explicit attention to the common good.

Bad Attitude

There are several special challenges to the use of this value framework in the
contemporary health care setting. The first, and in many ways the most significant, challenge is attitudinal. There is a rising sense of cynicism and even
hopelessness in the United States about social problems. Many health care
problems encountered in the emergency room, for example, are rooted in gang
violence, domestic abuse, homelessness, drug and alcohol addictions, and
automobile accidents.[33] Because these problems are all linked to individual

behavior and social conditions, they are theoretically preventable by personal decisions and social change. Yet the scope of these problems and the magnitude of the health care consequences are overwhelming. They seem to express deeply fixed habits and dysfunctions in American society. At the same time that the scale of these problems seems so daunting, many Americans have lost faith in the ability of public or private efforts to deal effectively with these problems. Cost overruns in existing programs, political corruption, and the inevitable tendency of past solutions to become part of contemporary problems reinforce the often expressed view that "government can't do anything right." Neither is there confidence that progress can be made by the private initiatives of corporations or voluntary associations. Thus, aside from exhortations to the individuals involved to come to grips with their own lives and take more personal responsibility, many Americans seem paralyzed by the nature of these problems.

As a result, there is considerable denial in American life. Intractable social problems are avoided as if they did not exist. The health care system has become a default safety net for many of the consequences of these problems. The emergency room is the only dependable social response to violence on our streets and highways. Neonatal intensive care units are filled with low-birth-weight babies whose mothers had no prenatal care and often have no husbands. Home health care agencies and visiting nurses grapple with health care problems intertwined with generations of welfare dependence and lack of opportunity. Hospitals are homes for "border babies" abandoned by their families because of HIV infection or crack addition or both. The health care system has many flaws, but it can hardly be held accountable for its inability to solve problems well out of its natural realm or for the costs associated with treating the health consequences of unaddressed social problems.

Viewed from the positive side, the value of service to the common good requires that attitudes of community and national solidarity be engendered. This means the development of feelings of caring and identification with those outside one's own immediate neighborhood, profession, and racial and ethnic groups. Ways must be found to tap, for these purposes, the same sort of solidarity that spontaneously generates in the face of warfare, national tragedies, or local disasters. In those cases, Americans look beyond divisions and think in terms of the interest of their entire local community or the nation itself. Unfortunately, when the war is over, the funeral ends, the flood recedes, people tend to go back to their private lives and shrug their shoulders at difficult social problems, relocating away from them, driving around them, and generally containing them by distance.

It is a difficult task to realign fundamental attitudes and to take on apparently insoluble problems, but it is imperative that ways of feeling and acting be developed to heal these serious fractures in our social relationships and institutions. Progress here will require multiple voluntary efforts of cultural regeneration. Inevitably, this will also require designing new government initiatives, many involving partnership with the private and voluntary sectors. Despite present cynicism, government (especially the federal government) remains one of the few organized endeavors in American life in which concern for the common good remains a natural language.

Prevention

Notwithstanding earlier cautions about abandoning the sick and dying as the health care system is reconstructed, it is plain that Americans need more stress on public health, health promotion, and disease prevention.[34] This need constitutes a second challenge in the area of the common good. By their very nature, public health efforts aim at the common good and are frequently chosen on the bases of frank utilitarian calculations; but these efforts also often have the potential for interfering with personal freedom. Gun control, motorcycle helmets, and smoke-free working environments are obvious cases in point. Because prizing freedom is also central to the common good, progress here means balancing competing values with care.

It is important to recall the dramatic successes of health education and prevention. There is a far greater awareness than ever before about the health implications of diet, cigarette smoking, alcohol abuse, etc. On smoking alone, there has been a dramatic change: An activity that was widely accepted only one or two generations ago has now become marginalized. Settings in which a large minority and even a majority of those present would have been smoking—in offices, restaurants, public meetings—now ban the conduct altogether. Success has been less dramatic for drug and alcohol use, but the cultural embedding of the notion of a designated driver is a victory of no small importance. Similar points can be made about nutrition awareness, the importance of regular exercise, containment of stress, etc. Americans have a long way to go before these battles are won, but it is important to realize how much has been done in how short a time.

More difficult than containing patterns of cigarette smoking are preventive measures that go to the heart of social structures. Preventing low-birth-weight babies, for example, and the high infant mortality associated with them require lifestyle changes that reach far beyond health promotion and education. Dealing with the cancers caused by industrial pollution, electromagnetic fields, and food processing requires difficult and expensive social change and will be resisted by powerful economic interests. Moreover, in the whole arena of public health, health promotion and preventive medicine, there is room for overreaching on the part of society that could undermine the value of human dignity, especially because so many of the issues involve matters of personal habits and privacy. Again, this is a matter for ongoing reappraisal. Yet in the present social environment, the imbalance still seems to lie with the individual, and more work needs to be done on behalf of the common good.

Priorities

A third special challenge to the value of the common good in the contemporary health care context lies in creating ways to involve the community in a meaningful dialogue about health care priorities. Although health care spending absorbs much of the national and local economies, there are few occasions when citizens can have any direct role in shaping the priorities of the system.

Operating under its own logic, the American health care system has become acute-care oriented, high-technology driven, and subspeciality dependent. These dispositions are exceptionally costly. The choice to invest considerable resources in organ transplantation, for example, is a choice to spend a great deal of money on a very few cases, just the opposite of what a utilitarian calculation would dictate. A community hospital with a world-class neonatal intensive care unit may also have a third-rate social work service, although the latter is cheaper and can often be instrumental in reducing the need for the former.

These momentous choices are not made and are seldom discussed in any public forum. Part of the reason for this is the pluralism of our health care system. Pieces of these decisions may have been made in a caucus room in the U.S. Congress or in the boardroom of a state Blue Cross program or at an administrative meeting of a private hospital or medical school. Moreover, all these decisions, even the public choices, are shaped to some extent by the competitive environment that has dominated the health care system over the last several decades and is becoming even more intense. When a voluntary, not-for-profit hospital considers whether to begin a new service, it must consider not only the need for the service in the community, but also the implications of adding the service for its competitive relations with other hospitals. Even in public programs, Medicare, for example, there is recognition that decisions shape and are shaped by competitive realities in the surrounding system. All this means there are few occasions when the health care common good is directly assessed and the citizenry is asked to help shape spending priorities. This is so despite the fact that the health care system is so heavily indebted to a social inheritance and to public funds.

One of the most positive signs in this arena is the development of the health decisions movement.[35] Under this rubric, many states have created multiple public fora in which citizens have articulated and prioritized their values and have attempted to influence the direction of health care policy. This model should be developed and used more often in states and in national decision-making.

Many citizens despair of these efforts because of the general distortion of communication and breakdown of trust across the nation. The resulting cynicism is a dangerous mood for a democracy that must rely on an educated and motivated citizenry. A recent experiment by political scientist James Fishkin offers new hope in this context.[36] Moved by the conviction that opinion polls and television represent the two worst aspects of American political culture, Fishkin has devised an ingenious response: Turn both technologies against their currently destructive tendencies. His experiment with technological democracy starts with a randomly selected representative group whose views on a given subject are polled. Unlike the bar graphs of contemporary politics, however, this group's opinions are the beginning, not the end, of discourse. These selected individuals are next brought together to interact with each other and with leaders in the substantive area under consideration, health care experts, for example. After three days of what amounts to an intensive seminar, the group then meets with leading politicians in a town hall format. The session is televised so that interactions between citizens and representatives are made public and their impact magnified. The result is a case study in educated democracy: a representative group of ordinary individuals who have examined the complexity of an issue and interacted publicly with their political leaders. Application of this model could help to expand and develop the health decisions movement and restore trust in democratic dialogue about social problems.

Finally, emphasis on the common good means developing a renewed sense of community. The notion of community is inherently vague and necessarily so. It is frequently given arbitrary boundaries for specific purposes: an urban community or a professional community. Yet it must be kept in mind that the notion itself, the idea of being-with-others, has *metaphysical* importance that goes beyond any arbitrary boundaries. It recalls the social nature of persons and underscores the fact that we participate, by chance or mysterious design, in a common human condition. We are here and now together, able to make experience better or worse for one another, and linked ineluctably whichever posture we choose. This is an especially important point to bear in mind as the United States cultivates a new sensitivity to diversity. Increased awareness of difference without an overarching sense of community can only mean increased social divisions. In the worst case, it can produce the nightmares of Beirut, Sarajevo, and Rwanda. Health care represents an opportunity to avoid these nightmares and to build community. It stands as a reminder of the core human realities that individuals share in common: pleasure and pain, happiness and suffering, life and death.

Community also extends through time so that deliberations about the common good must include reference to the needs of future generations as well as deference to the achievements and struggles of the past. It must also be remembered that national communities are themselves arbitrary. Although they have been the locus of great accomplishments and of dedicated patriotism, for centuries nations and nationalism have also been the root causes of warfare and other cruelty. The natural community of persons is not a nation, but the species itself. It is proper that citizens should fix their efforts immediately on the needs of their own nation's health care system, but the health care needs of suffering human beings around the world must be included in any comprehensive understanding of the common good.

Notes

1. Bellah et al. *Habits of the Heart*, pp. 142–163.
2. James Wetzel, "American Families: 75 Years of Change," *Monthly Labor Review* Vol. 113 no. 3 (March 1990): 4–13.
3. Harris and Wilkens, *Quiet Riots*.
4. Generally, see Jonathan Petrikin, *Male/Female Roles: Opposing Viewpoints* (San Diego, California: Greenhaven Press, 1995); and Steven Seidman, *Embattled Eros: Sexual Politics and Ethics in Contemporary America* (New York: Routledge, 1992).
5. Jethro Lieberman, *The Litigious Society* (New York: Basic Books, 1981).
6. On social psychology, see the classic work of George Herbert Mead, *Mind, Self, and Society*, ed. Charles Morris (Chicago: University of Chicago Press, 1965).
7. Paul Wise and DeWayne M. Pursey, "Infant Mortality as a Social Mirror," *The New England Journal of Medicine* 326, no. 23 (1992): 1558–60.
8. Ludwig Wittgenstein, *Philosophical Investigations*, trans. G. M. Anscombe (New York: Macmillan Company, 1968), no. 19, 23, and 241.
9. Michael Novak, *Free Persons and the Common Good* (New York: Madison Books, 1989), 21.
10. Marcus Raskin, *The Common Good* (New York: Routledge and Kegan Paul, 1986), 7–8.
11. Charles M. Sherover, *Time, Freedom, and the Common Good* (Albany: State University of New York Press, 1989), 6–9.
12. Committee for the Study of the Future of Public Health, *The Future of Public Health* (Washington, D.C.: National Academy Press, 1988), 56–72.
13. Aday, *At Risk in America*; James House, Karl Landis, and Debra Umberson, "Social Relationships and Health," *Science* 241 (July 29, 1988): 540–45.
14. See, e.g., Timothy McCoy, "Biomedical Process Patents: Should They be Restricted by Ethical Limitations?" *Journal of Legal Medicine* 13, no. 4 (1992): 501–19; Drummond Rennie, Annette Flanagen, and Richard Glass, "Conflicts of Interest in the Publication of Science," *JAMA* 266, no. 2 (1991): 266–67.
15. H. Gavaghan, "Genetics Business Booming Yet Uncertain," *Nature* 369, no. 6478 (1994): 341–2; and M. Leopold, "The Commercialization of Biotechnology," *Annals of the New York Academy of Science* 700 (December 21, 1993): 214–31;

Michael Witt and Lawrence Gostin, "Conflict of Interest Dilemmas in Biomedical Research," *JAMA* 271, no. 7 (1994): 547-51.

16. Paul Starr, *The Social Transformation of American Medicine* (New York: Basic Books, 1982), 348-51.

17. Ginsburg, *The Road to Reform*, pp. 14.

18. Starr, *Social Transformation of American Medicine*, pp. 308-34.

19. Dolenc and Dougherty, "DRGs: The Counterrevolution in Financing Health Care," pp. 19-29.

20. S. Christensen, "The Subsidy Provided Under Medicare to Current Enrollees," *Journal of Health Politics, Policy, and Law* 17, no. 2 (1992): 255-64.

21. Eckholm, *New York Times*, p. 22.

22. See, generally, J.C.C. Smart and Bernard Williams, eds., *Utilitarianism, For and Against* (Cambridge, Mass.: Cambridge University Press, 1973).

23. Dougherty, *American Health Care*, pp. 35-50.

24. John Stuart Mill, *On Liberty*, ed. David Spitz (New York: Norton, 1975), Chapter 1.

25. See, e.g., Joel Feinberg, "The Nature and Value of Rights," in Joel Feinberg, *Rights, Justice, and the Bounds of Liberty* (Princeton, N.J.: Princeton University Press, 1980), 143-155.

26. Charles J. Dougherty, "The Common Good, Terminal Illness, and Euthanasia" *Issues in Law and Medicine* 9, no. 2 (1993): 151-66.

27. James G. Randall, *Constitutional Problems Under Lincoln* (Urbana, Ill.: University of Illinois Press, 1964.)

28. Irving Howe, ed., *1984 Revisited: Totalitarianism in Our Century* (New York: Harper and Row, 1983).

29. Aristotle, *Nichomachean Ethics*, trans. Terence Irwin (Indianapolis, Ind.: Hackett Publishing Co., 1985), 49-52.

30. See, e.g., C. Sprung and B. Winick, "Informed Consent in Theory and Practice," *Critical Care Medicine* 17, no. 12 (1989): 1346-54.

31. Charles J. Dougherty, "Joined in Life and Death: On Separating the Lakeberg Twins," *Bioethics Forum* 11, no. 1 (1995): 9-16.

32. Arthur Caplan, Daniel Callahan, and Janet Haas, "Ethical and Policy Issues in Rehabilitation Medicine," *Hastings Center Report* Special Supplement (August 1987): 1-20; and Charles J. Dougherty, "Values in Rehabilitation: Happiness, Freedom, and Fairness," *Journal of Rehabilitation* (January/February/March 1991): 7-12.

33. J. Barber, "Telling the Public the Real Health Cost Story," *Hospitals* 66, no. 12 (1992): 68.

34. Dougherty, "Bad Faith and Victim-Blaming: The Limits of Health Promotion," pp. 111-119.

35. Bruce Jennings, "A Grassroots Movement in Bioethics," *Hastings Center Report* 18, no. 3 Supplement (1988): 1-16.

36. For some of the theoretical background, see James Fishkin, *Democracy and Deliberation: New Directions for Democratic Reform* (New Haven: Yale University Press, 1991). Fishkin described a practical application of this technique carried out in England at a meeting of the Communitarian Network in Los Angeles, California, on August 6, 1994.

7

Cost Containment

Foundations

There is no value named cost containment or even cost consciousness. Yet there is a value in the conceptual neighborhood of these terms that is exceptionally important in the contemporary health care arena. Whatever its proper name, its disposition is a kind of fiscal prudence. It might simply be called economics, had that term not lost its root meaning of efficient household management, an association still captured in the verb form, to economize.

The traditional moral value expressed in a desire to contain costs is thrift and under that name was long a central value for Americans.[1] It functioned as a value in several ways. Psychologically, thrift was valued as a form of puritan self-denial. It was an admired form of restraint that built character and self-sufficiency. The prizing of thrift has become such a foreign notion to contemporary Americans that both the name and the moral concept it expressed have all but disappeared from the culture in general and from discussions of ethics in particular. The closest contemporary expression of a value that celebrates self-denial is probably found in the areas of dieting and exercise, where restraint and self-discipline are still viewed positively, or at least seen to promote positive consequences.

Theoretically, thrift was also valued as an economic engine. At the same time that its psychology reduced demand, the financial dimensions of thrift produced savings. Americans who saved pennies put those pennies in banks. Thrift thus helped to create the capital needed for the development of modern economies, which in turn generated untold wealth. Before there was wealth, thrift also served as a practical means of coping with scarcity. In times of scarcity, the little available goes farther when all are thrifty with resources. Therefore, thrift was a value psychologically, economically, and practically.

This traditional stance began to wane in the United States after World War II. Practically, thrift was not needed in an economy of affluence and pent-up demand, nor was it the main economic engine; for individuals, corporations, and government borrowing replaced saving. The economic imperative of consumption fostered a psychological self-indulgence.

Large social trends, including the end of accelerating affluence, the increasing cost of debt, and the existential emptiness of consumerism, are beginning to move the nation back toward thrift. Americans are unlikely to embrace thrift as a moral value anytime soon, but there is an increasing moral repugnance toward waste. A move in this moral direction, away from waste and toward thrift, may introduce a greater balance in the national psyche and economy. The "golden mean" that lies between the two, at least in the arena of health care, is the value of cost containment.

The cost problem facing the American health care system has already been reviewed. The United States spends more on health care than any other nation in the world, more in dollars, more in terms of per capita spending, and more in terms of percentage of GDP. The rate of increase in spending is economically unsustainable. Projected into the near future, current rates will produce national spending of $1.7 trillion or 18.1 percent of the GDP, by the year 2000, $16 trillion or 32 percent of the GDP by 2030.[2]

This economic perspective is challenging enough on its own terms, but the need to contain costs in the health care system is also a moral issue for three reasons. First, if the health care needs of the American people can be met by spending less money, other things being equal, this should be done. Reversing the point, spending more money than necessary to address the health care needs of the population is wasteful. It is easy to be cynical on this point because what constitutes waste to one person is often income to another. Nevertheless, besides the growing cultural hostility toward it, there is a common sense moral prohibition against wastefulness. Although Americans in the second half of the twentieth century have been inclined to ignore or minimize this moral prohibition, it has become increasingly clear that the twenty-first century will be an era of limits.[3] The kind of limits that have shaped the characters of other nations and other times—limits on space, resources, financing, even opportunity—are now coming forward in the American conscious-ness. These limits are being reached politically by the reluctance of the public to approve new spending measures and programs, being defined in the market-place by the increasing reluctance of payers to absorb rising health care costs, and being experienced in many households as more of the costs of health care are shifted to consumers. At the same time that limits are becoming increas-ingly irresistible, growth in the health care sector since World War II has made it one of the largest economic activities in the United States. In many Ameri-can cities and towns, for example, hospitals are the largest employers and the largest consumers of resources. These facts have heightened awareness of the need to contain costs and given new urgency to the general moral wrongful-ness of waste.

A parallel point can be made in religious terms drawn from the Judeo–Christian tradition.[4] Creation and all its multiple resources are gifts from a benevolent God, given in trust to the human species as part of a redemptive plan that is understood only "through a glass darkly." Because of the richness of the gift of nature and the incomprehensible character of the full plan for its intended use, the religious tradition has given rise, especially in modern industrial nations, to exploitative attitudes toward nature and other species. Selfishness and the drive to dominate have led to cruelties, pollution, and a generalized indifference to the issue of waste. Although these cultural expres-sions arose within the Judeo–Christian tradition, they do not embody its more fundamental religious insight: the duty of responsible stewardship.[5] The main intellectual thrust of the tradition is that humans are not given control over nature for purposes of domination and self-aggrandizement, but for working out a partnership in the creative work of God. In this view, waste can never simply be an economic matter. Instead, it is a profound disorientation from the basic gift of creation. Waste constitutes an act of ingratitude to God. The main thrust of the dominant religious tradition therefore supports the same conclusion as common sense: If the health care needs of the American people can be met while spending less, it should be done.

Opportunity Costs

A second reason why cost containment is a moral issue involves the economic notion of opportunity costs. There are at least two aspects of cost to purchas-ing any good or service. The first cost is the money spent directly for the item. Less obvious perhaps, but nonetheless real, is the indirect cost entailed by the fact that the money spent on this item is no longer available to be spent in any other fashion. Thus a purchaser pays the direct cost for an item and pays again indirectly in lost opportunities to purchase other items. The United States now invests one-seventh of all spending in the health care sector.[6] Not only is this a staggeringly large figure in its own right (approaching one trillion dollars), but it also represents money not available for spending elsewhere, including areas in which there are significant unmet needs.[7]

The impact of these opportunity costs can be seen most graphically in state government. For a number of years, the item growing most rapidly in the budgets of most states has been the Medicaid program.[8] Total costs of the program (federal and state) more than doubled between 1989 and 1993. Medicaid costs to the states have exploded because of growing numbers of uninsured and those using the program for longterm care.

In many states this massive increase in Medicaid spending has substantially diminished discretionary spending by the state, that is, reduced the state's ability to initiate new efforts in other areas of pressing need. States have been less able, for example, to improve the lives and lots of their own citizens through initiatives in social welfare, economic development, housing, and education. There is considerable irony in this. One of the obvious goals of health care is to preserve and enhance the health of the population and individuals who constitute the population. (It must always be recalled that caring, irrespective of state of health or anticipated outcome, is also a goal of health care.) Interventions in these other areas, especially in education, housing, and economic development, can make dramatic differences in a population's health and, of course, in the health of individuals.[9] Consequently, one of the opportunity costs of an ever-expanding health care sector is the inability to improve health through non-health-care efforts.

Finally, cost containment is a moral value because waste in this arena often means the performance of unnecessary procedures. When too much money is spent on health care, too many interventions are done. A recent study, for example, suggests that twenty-three percent of procedures to place tympanostomy tubes in children (for otitis media or ear infections) are inappropriate, and another thirty-five percent are questionable.[10] Too many interventions means the creation of harms through unnecessary surgery and invasive tests. Whereas it is plainly imperative from a moral point of view to get people the health care that they need, it is also imperative for similar reasons not to provide health care people do not need, especially risky health care. Yet this obvious point can easily be lost in an overheated and intensely competitive economic sector that may soon absorb one of every five dollars in the United States economy.

Rationing

There are, therefore, good reasons for moral concern about health care spending and for commitment to the goals of restraining cost increases and avoiding waste in the system. On the other hand, the need to create universal coverage grounded in the fundamental value of dignity is also clear. There may be other strategies for balancing the apparently incompatible demands of increasing access while restraining costs, but one is surely the rationing of health care. Debates on this subject have been extraordinarily complex and heated. Honesty demands that the ethical dimensions of this debate be treated straightforwardly and with care.[11]

Part of the reason the debate about health care rationing has been so acrimonious is because the meaning of the term is equivocal when applied to health care, and differing meanings are associated with directly antagonistic emotional evaluations.[12] One side, typically held by direct providers of care, understands rationing to be the denial of needed health care services in clinical contexts. A sinister image that typically operates behind this understanding is a scenario in which a doctor tries to help a patient whose life can be saved or whose illness can be cured by access to an available but expensive technology. Standing between the doctor and patient, however, and preventing the ability of the former to assist the latter is a government bureaucrat. This functionary refuses authorization to use the machine on the basis of some estimation of the total cost of such interventions to society as a whole. Thus, the clinical point of medicine and the satisfactions of both provider and patient are frustrated by health care rationing. More importantly, the patient is harmed and may die unnecessarily or suffer a preventable loss of health. Therefore, from this perspective, rationing means denying needed care, and its emotional association is exceptionally negative. Rationing is wrong and should be resorted to only in the most grave and unusual circumstances, for example, in situations of triage caused by large-scale disasters.

There is, however, a competing interpretation of rationing, a view typically held by social workers, economists, and policy experts. In this view, rationing is an inevitable dimension of economic life, a means of allocating resources. Moreover, in some circumstances, it can be a means morally preferable to other alternatives. This view gets semantic support from dictionaries in which rationing is often defined as the *equitable* distribution of a scarce resource.[13] In this context, equitable simply means fair. Therefore, rationing means the introduction of fairness into a situation of scarcity. Because scarcity is itself an inevitable phenomena—there is rarely an unlimited amount of any desirable resource—rationing creates the opportunity to bring fairness into economic relationships. By contrast, the unhampered workings of a market system tend to drive the price of scarce commodities up, to the point that only the wealthiest can afford to buy them. This seems unfair and can be destructive of a community's sense of solidarity. Rationing assures that wealth is not the sole criteria for access to scarce commodities. It therefore makes the economic situation fairer than the pricing system on its own would be and thus prevents social discord. Rationing of health care has similar potential for creating greater fairness in the distribution of an inevitably scarce set of goods and services and for expressing national solidarity. Emotionally, this account of rationing feels good.

A Definition

To move beyond this impasse in both meaning and emotional charge, it is necessary to stipulate a neutral definition of rationing. It should be one comprehensive enough to include the valid insights of both sides, yet one that does not determine by definition that all forms of rationing are inherently either good or bad. The following definition is employed here. *Health care rationing is the denial or limiting of access to needed and potentially beneficial health care because policies and practices have restricted the resources available for health care.*[14]

This neutral definition captures valid points made by both sides of the debate. On the one hand, it recognizes that rationing does mean the denial of needed health care. On the other hand, it allows that policies and practices must sometimes be shaped around the facts of scarcity. It does not, however, assume by definition that rationing as such is a good thing. This neutral definition does not entail, as many dictionary definitions do, that all schemes of rationing are fair by making equity a defining property of rationing. To reach a moral evaluation, particular schemes of rationing would have to be analyzed on their own terms. Some arrangements may be fair, others unfair. Therefore, criteria are needed by which actual or proposed rationing policies and practices can be evaluated morally. Before elaborating such criteria, one other important aspect of this definition should be detailed and more said about the general ethical challenge of rationing.

This is a broad definition. As such, it makes evident what too often escapes contemporary commentators, namely, that there is a considerable amount of rationing in the health care system at present. For the millions of uninsured, health care is limited to emergency treatment and by the charity of providers. For those in public programs, access is rationed by determination of the basic benefits package and by the eligibility standards of the programs themselves. There are, for example, very rigorous norms for financial eligibility for Medicaid in many states, and some are getting more restrictive. There is rationing, too—a peculiar form of it—in the fact that a poor sixty-four-year-old with desperate health care needs may have no health insurance in the United States, whereas every sixty-five-year-old is covered by Medicare, irrespective of need or income. There is rationing in private health plans. Limitations on services covered, maximum days of service allowed, and dollar caps all establish restrictions on access for beneficiaries.

Other features of the system also work to restrict or deny access to needed health care and thus constitute forms, however subtle, of rationing. Geography can be a significant barrier to care in many rural parts of the United States. Lack of infrastructure, difficulties in transportation, and cultural and linguistic differences create barriers for many living in American inner cities. Consequently, de facto rationing occurs in the health care system at present, much of it quite unconscious and unintended, some of it planned.[15] Hence a complete moral evaluation of any proposal to ration health care must analyze not only the details of the health care rationing proposal itself, but must also compare it with the rationing in place in the system at present. It may well be that some rationing proposals have significant moral flaws but compared with the present situation would constitute improvements. In these cases, prudence must be used to determine whether more explicit and formal kinds of rationing are preferable to the indirect and unspoken rationing that permeates the present system.

It is also important to detail the general moral problems raised by rationing health care. The most obvious problem is contained in the first portion of the definition. If health care rationing means the denial of or limitation of access to needed care, then rationing can hurt people. People may be disappointed or frustrated by the inability to obtain unnecessary or futile care, but lack of access to *needed* care means serious harms. Compared with the hypothetical possibility of a system that provides unlimited access to all needed health care, a rationed system means the acceptance of preventable death and suffering. Specific proposals to ration health care, however, must be compared not with this hypothetical ideal, but to the rationing already in place in the system. Some proposals to ration care may involve new harms or new distributions of existing harms, or they may remove or lessen existing harms. Despite the necessity for it and the other positive things that might be said in favor of a thoughtful and comprehensive plan of rationing, from the point of view of the individual denied needed health care, rationing creates real harms. It is important to stress that these harms are not equivalent to those created when commodities like gasoline or sugar are rationed, but can literally mean the difference between life and death and the difference between significant degrees of health for real individuals.

Easy Rescue

Another significant ethical issue raised by health care rationing is the possibility that it may violate the general moral duty to come to the aid of those in need. This duty is real, but its scope must be limited.[16] Human needs are endless. Moreover, persons have fundamental liberties as well as moral duties to others. Therefore, some reasonable boundaries must exist to the duty to aid those in need. One strategy for charting boundaries here is by understanding the duty to aid as one of "easy rescue." On this account, the duty to rescue others is morally compelling only when three conditions are present. First, a substantial benefit can be conferred on those in need or a substantial harm to them avoided. Second, the risk of harm to the would-be rescuer is insignificant or at least substantially less than the benefit at stake for those in need. Finally, the would-be rescuer must be practically capable, acting alone or with others, to effect the rescue. On this account, people are not obligated, for example, to place their lives in jeopardy to secure a minor benefit for another. However, when an individual or a group is able at a small risk to save the life of another, then it is morally incumbent on them to try, hence the notion of a moral obligation of "easy rescue."

If there is an obligation to provide easy rescue, then health care rationing may violate that duty if it denies substantial benefits to those in need when these benefits could be provided without great harm to others. Put in more general terms, there is an obligation to provide some basic level of health care to others if this can be done at a reasonable cost. Rationing could violate this duty, and surely some present forms of rationing do violate it.

Finally, depending on how a rationing scheme is designed, it may, dictionary definitions notwithstanding, create inequities in access to health care. Rationing of health care could be based on invidious or inappropriate criteria. For example, denying health care on the basis of general intelligence, strength, or membership in a given race or ethnic group would satisfy the general definition of rationing but would at the same time introduce new and substantial inequities into the distribution of health care. Moreover, certain of these inequities, especially those having to do with racial discrimination, would create with them indignities that undermine respect for persons in substantial ways. Thus, the direct harms created inevitably by rationing— denial of needed care—may under some plans be compounded by indirect harms of inequity and indignity.

With these considerations in mind, eight criteria are useful in helping to determine whether an existing or proposed system of rationing is ethically acceptable.[17] In an area so morally complex, these criteria are not meant to serve as a checklist, nor are the criteria to be thought of in quantitative terms. It would be wrong to think, for example, that a rationing scheme satisfying six of the eight criteria is acceptable, whereas one satisfying only five of the eight is not. Moral evaluation is inherently more ambiguous and difficult than that. These criteria are offered rather as eight moral considerations that should be raised in the evaluation of the ethical acceptability of a rationing plan. They must be used with practical wisdom. The first four of the eight criteria follow more or less directly from values that have already been articulated in previous chapters.

Cover Everyone

1. *Rationing should take place only in a system that provides a basic level of care for everyone.* The value of human dignity and its expression in respect for persons provide the basis for this criterion. The connection to rationing is that it would be unfair and would create indignities to develop a rationing scheme for health care when some people in effect would have access to nothing more than emergency treatment. Putting the point affirmatively, it is important to bring everyone into the system and to structure a health care floor before the limitations on the system, the ceiling, can be reasonably and fairly determined.

Obviously, determination of what counts as a basic benefit package already involves rationing choices. To exclude bone marrow transplant, for example, because it is too expensive to provide to everyone who might benefit from it (or too expensive in light of serious dispute about its benefits) means that some people who might benefit, might have their lives extended meaningfully, from this procedure will face the harms of being denied it. This sort of rationing choice is inherent in any determination of a basic benefit package. The situation is therefore not as simple as creating universal coverage and then facing the need to ration. Rationing choices are made in the determination of the basic benefits to be provided to all. Nonetheless, the moral imperative is clear: Fairness requires that everyone have some before the limits are determined for all.

Preserve Caring and Trust

2. *Health care rationing must preserve the intangibles of caring and trust.* As argued above, caring is at the heart of the project of health care and trust in individual health care providers and in the professions in general is a significant aspect of maintaining caring relationships. Health care rationing has the potential for undermining both. The need for rationing represents a frank recognition of fiscal and political limits. It arises at a time when cost-cutting methods are becoming increasingly ruthless. Consequently, there is a possibility that explicit rationing may further undermine the climate of caring. It may make the economic dimensions of health care so insistent that the intangibles associated with altruism are driven out. Moreover, concrete expressions of care are often expensive. The ratio of nurses to hospital inpatients, for example, or the number of hospice professionals available for home care of the dying can make a significant difference in a patient's experience of care. Yet labor costs are some of the most expensive items in the health care system. Unlike the relatively fixed costs of building and equipment, labor costs

are also variable, reducible by program and staff cuts. Assessment of the moral acceptability of rationing must make reference to protection of caring even as responsible limits on health care are set explicitly.

Depending on how health care rationing is organized, there is also a potential for undermining trust in providers of care, especially in doctors. Suppose, for example, that doctors were asked to become agents of rationing schemes in health care plans, perhaps by managing a given amount of resources for a number of enrolled individuals. In such a scheme, services provided to one patient could mean services not available to another. Doctors in this situation would have to consider not only whether a given patient needs a service, but also whether other potential patients in the health care plan will have a greater need for the service within the same fiscal period. This kind of financial assessment has the potential for developing conflicts of interest in the primary fiduciary relationship between doctor and patient. It can pit an individual patient's interests against the hypothetical interests of other patients. From the patient's point of view, this introduces an element of distrust. A patient could have a reasonable worry that a doctor's advice that a procedure is unnecessary or unavailable is motivated by a desire to save the procedure for another patient, perhaps one who is more compliant or who has a more interesting case. This, of course, is an insidious concern that can erode trust in the doctor–patient relationship.

The specific role of doctors and other direct care providers in rationing health care services is a complex and controversial one, but assessment of the moral acceptability of a rationing schemes must begin with the premise that some forms of doctor involvement will be incompatible with the trust they must preserve with their patients. Doctors can provide important advice about health care rationing at the policy level and must therefore have a leading role in public debates on rationing. In clinical settings, however, it is better to have rationing imposed on doctors and patients by policymakers and administrators. In this way, doctors can remain advocates for their patients, fighting the bureaucrats who arrange and enforce the limitations.

Protect the Vulnerable

3. *Rationing must protect the most vulnerable among us.* As argued above, there is a special obligation to protect those who are least able to protect themselves. Health care rationing represents a conscious recognition of the struggle over scarce resources in which some will be able to bring greater influence on their own behalf, whereas some will be less able to do so. Children, the frail elderly, the mentally and physically disabled, and those subject

to discrimination may find themselves disadvantaged in rationing arrangements unless their case is defended strongly by others who are able to do so.

Defending the interests of the vulnerable may have to take the form of affirmative action. If a rationing scheme were to accept the present distribution of health care resources and to place caps on it without fundamental reallocation, then inner cities, rural areas, Indian reservations, and other areas would face special additional hardships. Within the general restrictions central to the development of a rationing scheme, there must be sufficient flexibility so that additional resources can be directed to historically underserved areas.

Serve the Common Good

4. *Rationing schemes must serve the common good.* This criterion follows from the social nature of persons and of the health care system and from the general moral importance of community. It means, for example, that some expensive procedures that benefit only a few, even life-saving treatments, must be foregone in favor of health care investments that make a greater difference statistically. This is an application of the utilitarian dimension of the common good: the greatest good for the greatest number.

This criterion will not be easy to apply. Some investments in expensive medical technology, for example, may serve the overall interests of a community in the long run because the technology becomes cheaper over time or leads to discoveries that benefit all. On the other hand, explicit rationing must begin by assuring access to garden-variety health care of the sort that makes a significant difference in the community as a whole: prenatal care, pediatrics, comprehensive emergency services, and other services. Applying this simple point to the U.S. health care system would entail great change. Current tendencies favor high-tech, acute-care interventions for individuals over public health measures that could make some dramatic differences in the overall health of communities. The facts suggest that Americans prefer spending extravagantly on neonatal intensive care for low-birth-weight babies, for example, while begrudging funding for the relatively inexpensive educational and nutritional efforts that could surely reduce the incidence of low birth weight and infant mortality. Recent and proposed cuts in social programs and welfare have exacerbated this balance.

Use of this criterion also presents an occasion for detailed consideration of the opportunity costs of increased spending throughout the health care sector. If the overall health of the community could be improved by shifting some investments from health care to social services, education, housing, and economic development, then this should be done.

Rationing Must Be Necessary

5. *Health care rationing must be necessary.* At first glance, this may seem an easy criterion to satisfy. The point has already been made that expanding access while simultaneously containing costs requires rationing. Therefore, the general necessity of rationing is easily established; but in a system as complex as the American health care system, there are many layers and cross currents of rationing. At present, for example, rationing choices are made in private insurance companies, at the federal level in the Medicare program, and at the state level in the Medicaid program. If all these choices were made consciously and explicitly, some of the rationing implications would be seen as necessary, but others would not be. For example, it may well be that federal spending on health care is approaching its political limits. It is far less clear, however, that all the states are putting adequate money into their Medicaid systems.[18] Some of the rationing by private insurers and by managed care plans is justified only by considerations of the corporate "bottom line."

To determine the necessity for any specific scheme of rationing inside the total system of American health care, difficult practical questions must be asked. Is the proper amount of money being put into that area of health care? The need for rationing in cancer care, for example, might be made more or less pressing depending on how much money is spent on AIDS research and vice versa. In addition to questions involving the internal distribution of health care resources, larger questions arise about how much is put into the entire system and by whom. Is fifteen percent of the GDP the right amount to be spending on health care? Is twenty percent? Are states paying their fair share? What is the proper role of private employers, individual taxpayers, and providers themselves? Assessment of the need for rationing must begin with examination of whether all these players contribute their appropriate share.

The issue of waste is pertinent here as well. Health care rationing, especially the kind that results in significant harms for individuals, is very hard to justify in light of the apparent waste in the system. Imagine a family being told that a rationing arrangement has disqualified their child from an expensive but potentially life-saving intervention. Heart-wrenching scenarios like this will occur in any serious rationing scheme; they occur now. Suppose, further, that after being denied this care because it is too expensive, the same family discovers the amount of money health care providers put into advertising each year, the high salaries paid to executives throughout the system, or the profits made by pharmaceutical companies. How can this hypothetical family understand and accept the life and death restrictions they face once they know the costs of the many unnecessary medical procedures performed each year, the extraordinary amount of administrative overhead in the system, or the stock market profits of investors in for-profit health care corporations?

This criterion does not require that every form of waste be removed from the system before rationing can be justified. This would be an impossible standard. It does mean, however, that it becomes more difficult to justify rationing as there is more obvious waste in the system. There can be considerable differences in opinion about what constitutes waste in health care, and these differences must be respected. One obvious benchmark is the amount of money spent outside the context of patient care. The further health care spending is from patient care, the higher the standard for justifying its use. Rationing means asking for shared sacrifice. A plausible case must be made that this level of sacrifice is indeed required. Every bit of waste makes the case that much less plausible.

Keep the Process Open

6. *Health care rationing must result from an open public process.* Everyone affected by rationing must have access to the process through which the limits are set. This access may occur through the political process, for example, through public hearings, legislation, and candidates for election debating explicit rationing goals and methods. This criterion also requires opening the rationing processes of private entities to public scrutiny. Enrollees should be able to know, for example, the reasons why an insurance company determines that bone marrow transplantation is not covered, why an HMO covers only thirty days of care in a rehabilitation hospital, why a managed care plan reduced its mental health care benefits. Enrollees should have some ways to shape these decisions. Many members of the public will not be able to understand the complexities of medical outcome studies and actuarial determinations of risk and service utilization. Some will have no interest in influencing coverage decisions. Nonetheless, all citizens should have access to the process that sets specific limitations on their care as a matter of rudimentary fairness. If the sacrifices of rationing are to be shared, there must be some ownership of the process that determines the specific character of the sacrifice. Fairness also requires easy access to unbiased appeals processes for individuals who are denied the health care they need.

No Discrimination

7. *Health care rationing must be free of wrongful discrimination.* Obviously, health care rationing means discriminating between covered and uncovered services and between individuals who are and are not candidates for services. Some choices may appear unfair from some individuals' points of view, espe-

cially those denied needed care. Nevertheless, this sort of discrimination is a requirement of health care rationing; it is what health care rationing means.

At the same time, however, health care rationing must be free of invidious forms of discrimination, including discrimination based on gender, race, ethnicity, religion, medical condition or disability, sexual orientation, etc. As difficult as enforcement may be on these issues, the moral point behind them is obvious to most Americans. However, there are two other areas in which consensus is more elusive.

The first area is age.[19] From one point of view, the use of age as a way to ration health care is as unacceptable as the use of race or gender. From this viewpoint, denying people medical procedures because they are elderly constitutes ageism. This view does embody a sound insight, namely, that consideration of age alone is a morally arbitrary criterion. Furthermore, it is a criterion that discriminates against a population that is generally both vulnerable because of the natural effects of aging and deserving because of a lifetime of contributions to society.

Yet age is unlike other clearly discriminatory categories in one important respect. As a rule, people do not change their gender or race. By contrast, people change their age with predictable regularity. A policy that links health care benefits to age so that certain benefits are available only after a given age (mammography, for example) and others available only before a given age (immunizations, for example) could be fair. Such a policy would affect people equally, not at the same time, but equally as they move through time. It is not unfair, broadly speaking, that more educational resources are invested on the young and more health care on the elderly because this distribution captures part of the natural rhythm of life in the contemporary world. From this perspective, age-based criteria for rationing are not inherently discriminatory. Instead, they can be reasonable patterns of social support for temporal beings.

One strategy for resolving this tension, especially as it bears on the very expensive care of the elderly and dying, is to restrict the use of age as a criterion for rationing to its relationship to prognosis. It seems discriminatory, for example, to deny seventy-year-olds heart transplantation simply because of their age, but it does seem reasonable to exclude them if patients over seventy have a demonstrably lower chance of success from such procedures. There are contexts in which this is not an easy distinction to make, nor will it be fair to all people since some seventy-year-olds will be more robust and therefore have a better individual prognosis than their age cohort. Yet the need for rationing is such that age is a reasonable consideration when it is clearly related to medical outcome, but not otherwise.

The other unsettling dimension of potential discrimination in this area is rationing based on lifestyle, especially when it involves alleged complicity in the etiology of disease. Is it fair, for example, to restrict access to certain treatments for emphysema when this condition was caused by lifelong cigarette smoking at the same time that these same treatments are available to others who have non-smoking–related emphysema?

It is important to ask individuals to assume more responsibility for their health and health care. It makes sense to use financial incentives and disincentives to encourage positive habits and discourage others. However, the use of notions of personal responsibility in the context of need for care can easily devolve into "victim-blaming."[20] This is especially so in light of the fact that the multiple variables that shape habit—genetics, environment, personal choice—are so interwoven as to make assessment of degree of responsibility a practically impossible task. Moreover, using personal responsibility to determine access to care could undermine the caring attitude so necessary for health care professionals and institutions.

On balance, then, individuals should be presumed responsible when prevention and health education efforts are mounted. Some financial incentives can be acceptable. In clinical context, however, it is inappropriate to use lifestyle or personal responsibility for health in making rationing decisions. Here a caring response to patient need is the right attitude, not judgmental and debatable assessments of responsibility.

Rationing for All

8. *Those who ration health care should be subject to rationing themselves.* This is at once the most obvious and the most challenging criterion. It is the most obvious because of the evident unfairness in allowing a system in which some people ration health care for others and yet remain free of the same restrictions that they create. The state legislators who vote to restrict access to Medicaid, but who have comprehensive coverage for themselves, are a case in point. So is the case of the U.S. Senator who opposes universal health care coverage but receives publicly funded comprehensive care. The Golden Rule, an insight at the core of many religious and ethical codes, mandates that one adopt the same standards of conduct toward others that one would want were roles reversed. The Golden Rule insight demands moral reciprocity. It disallows making exceptions for oneself, rejecting as immoral, for example, an insistence on honesty from others but on freedom to lie for oneself. Yet this is the same kind of moral exception claimed, in effect, by "unrationed rationers." These people and their families enjoy access to all that contemporary health care can offer, while at the same time they limit—actively or passively—access for others. On the face of it, this is inequitable. It creates a kind of medical class system.

On the other hand, the reason this principle is so difficult to accept and apply has to do with the plural character of the U.S. health care system. The state legislator, for example, who votes to restrict access to services in the Medicaid program may have Blue Cross insurance coverage provided by a private employer. As a state legislator, this person is placing restrictions on the spending of public funds; as a private citizen, this same person is accepting a fringe benefit in a private employment contract.

Demanding that those who ration be subject to the rationing they impose would be more feasible were the system more unitary. For example, if there were a national health board that determined the basic benefit package for all Americans, it would be a reasonable demand that the individuals who determine that package live with it themselves. The practical expectation is that the standards for acceptable rationing would rise when rationing is also applied to the rationers and their families, not simply to "the other." Yet this anticipates large and complex changes in the health care system.

Moreover, this criterion runs into another fundamental American value, the freedom to accumulate and dispose of wealth. Suppose some member of the national commission that determines the basic benefit package to be provided to all is a corporate leader and a millionaire. It would violate fundamental assumptions in American culture to forbid this individual from using some personal wealth to purchase additional health care beyond the minimal package designed by the board. It certainly seems problematic to hold that a millionaire can own multiple homes, cars, and endless luxury items but cannot buy more dialysis or better long-term care.

For these reasons, a more pragmatic version of the same principle would require movement toward a health care system that has such a comprehensive basic benefit package that even well-off citizens (though perhaps not the truly wealthy) would have little inclination to buy more, or at least those who did would be few. These considerations raise the problem of a two-tiered or multitiered health care system. A strict interpretation of the principle that those who ration must be subject to rationing anticipates a unitary system with one tier of care for all. This may never be the case in the United States. If one tier is never to be, the nature of the tiers that are probable must be assessed because some tier arrangements are morally preferable to others.

A system with fewer people in a second, more comprehensive tier of care is morally better than one with a large percentage of the population in a second, better tier. For example, a situation in which ten percent of the population buys more than the basic benefit package is morally preferable to a situation in which seventy-five percent of the population buys more. In the second scenario, there is good reason to think that what is defined as basic in the benefit package is inadequate; certainly the majority behaves as if they believe it is so. Moreover, with so many people buying more or relying on a different system entirely, there would be little political support to keep the quality high and the benefit package adequate in the publicly defined system. Consequently, a practical compromise with the realities of the American health care system now and in the foreseeable future requires a moral strategy that seeks to keep as many of the powerful and influential rationers, especially middle class voters, in a single system of rationing. Inevitably, some Americans will have the desire and ability to escape health care restrictions by using their own private funds. As troubling as this compromise is from the Golden Rule perspective, it is built around presently irreducible facts about the nation's political culture.

The logic of recent debates on health care rationing has been disingenuous on both sides. Progressives who demand universal access insist at the same time that expansion of access has no connection to the need for health care rationing; this is false. Health care rationing is probably the only tool available for achieving the twin goals of expanded access and cost constraint. At the same time, conservatives who resist demands for universal access invoke the specter of health care rationing as if restrictions would occur only under some new scheme for universal coverage, as if there were no rationing in the present system; this is also false. The health care system rations now. Issues of rationing are unavoidable either way. There is rationing in American health care now. There will be rationing in American health care in any conceivable future. The real question is whether ethical criteria will be used to guide it.

Notes

1. David M. Tucker, *The Decline of Thrift in America* (New York: Praeger, 1991).
2. Sally Burner, Daniel Waldo, and David McKusick, "National Health Expenditures Projections Through 2030," *Health Care Financing Review* 14, no. 1 (1992): 1-30.
3. Callahan, *Setting Limits*.
4. On Christianity and the environment, see John Carmody, *Ecology and Religion: Toward a New Christian Theology of Nature* (New York: Paulist Press, 1983); and James M. Gustafson, *A Sense of the Divine: The Natural Environment from a Theocentric Perspective* (Cleveland, Ohio: Pilgrim Press, 1994).
5. Prentiss Pemberton, *Toward a Christian Economic Ethic: Stewardship and Social Power* (Minneapolis: Winston Press, 1985); and Mary Evelyn Jegen and Bruno Manno, eds., *The Earth is the Lord's: Essays on Stewardship* (New York: Paulist Press, 1978).
6. Eckholm, *New York Times,* pp. 1 and 20.
7. Ibid.
8. Iglehart, "Medicaid," pp. 896-900.
9. See, e.g., E. Rogot P. Sorlie, N. Johnson, "Life Expectancy by Employment Status, Income, and Education in the National Longitudinal Mortality Study," *Public Health Reporter* 107, no. 4 (1992): 457-61.

10. L. Kleinman, et al., "The Medical Appropriateness of Tympanostomy Tubes Proposed for Children Younger Than 16 Years in the United States," *JAMA* 271, no. 16 (1994): 1250–55.
11. Charles J. Dougherty, *Ethical Dimensions of Healthcare Rationing*, (St. Louis, Catholic Health Association, 1994), 1–13.
12. Larry Churchill, *Self Interest and Universal Health Care* (Cambridge, Mass.: Harvard University Press, 1994), 6–23.
13. See, e.g., *Webster's Ninth New Collegiate Dictionary* (Springfield, Mass.: Merriam-Webster, 1983), 977.
14. Dougherty, "Ethical Dimensions of Healthcare Rationing," p. 3.
15. Larry R. Churchill, *Rationing Health Care in America* (Notre Dame, Ind.: University of Notre Dame Press, 1987), 5–19.
16. Beauchamp and Childress, *Principles of Biomedical Ethics*, pp. 266–71.
17. Dougherty, "Ethical Dimensions of Healthcare Rationing," pp. 8–13.
18. Marilyn Bach et al., "Ethics and Medicaid: A New Look at an Old Problem," *Journal of Health Care for the Poor and Underserved* 2, no. 4 (1992), pp. 427–47.
19. See, generally, Norman Daniels, *Am I My Parents' Keeper?* (New York: Oxford University Press, 1988), esp. pp. 83–102.
20. Charles J. Dougherty, "Bad Faith and Victim-Blaming: The Limits of Health Promotion," *Health Care Analysis* 1, no. 3, (1993): 111–19.

8

Responsibility

Foundations

A key value that lies at the heart of many health care debates is the notion of responsibility. It is a part of our moral common sense that freedom entails responsibility. When someone or some group has a range of authority or certain rights, it is appropriate to hold that individual or group accountable for the exercise of that authority or those rights. It is a natural inclination, for example, when encountering a mistake or a problem, to attempt to determine whose decision or negligence led to the difficulty. This can be done for educational reasons or to identify who has the primary responsibility for correcting the problem. It can also result in blaming or punishing those responsible. For several reasons, this natural part of our secular consciousness is undergoing considerable change, often making the notion of responsibility difficult to understand and to employ. There are also practical limits to the application of this notion to individuals in clinical contexts.

Yet the idea of responsibility is a simple and unavoidable aspect of moral common sense. Praise and blame are linked to responsibility, neither making sense without it. Both the praiseworthy and the blameworthy (generally competent adults) are in a world of morality, a world composed of good and bad, right and wrong. Everyone and everything else exists in a nonmoral world, including young children, animals, and natural events. In a moral world, agents are responsible for what *ought to be*. Events in a nonmoral world without responsibility just happen. This world can and should be valued by moral agents; beings without responsibility still have intrinsic worth, but they cannot be held accountable. They are not moral peers. With responsibility, however, comes the potential for all the mutual relations of equals. In a nonmoral world without responsibility, there is no reciprocal "gratitude, resentment, forgiveness, anger, friendship, and love."[1] All these moral judgments and relationships of responsibility turn on assessments of a person's character, the capacities or habits of conduct that grow through use and allow reasonable predictions about how an individual will behave. "She is trustworthy" and "He is dishonest" are judgments of moral responsibility grounded in assessments of a person's character, of how they have acted and likely will act. They are also acknowledgments of a shared moral world.

There are various kinds of responsibility. In addition to personal responsibility (he did it), there is also role responsibility (she is accountable for that).[2] The most primitive role responsibility is parental, an emotionally strong yet diffuse responsibility. Parents are responsible for everything for young children. A more focused (but typically less passionate) responsibility is that of a social role: "The physiatrist is responsible for the rehabilitation plan." More focused yet is the voluntary assumption of responsibility: "I will treat that patient." All these cases of role responsibility are linked to personal responsibility. Persons are held responsible for activities for which they are accountable. In every case, assessment of the degree of responsibility, of how much of an act truly reflects a person's character, is based on the degree of understanding the agent had (or should have had) about the situation, the ability the agent had to project the likely consequences of alternative choices, and the real power of the agent to affect events, to choose alternatives. Since each of these factors has increased in the twentieth century (more information, more planning, and more power), it is appropriate that contemporaries be held to higher standards of responsibility than earlier generations. Because we understand the causes and effects of pollution and have more ability to control them, we are more accountable for them. Because we know the health consequences of various lifestyles and presumably can alter them, we can be held more responsible for their effects.

It is easy to identify the roots of this bit of moral common sense in the dominant religious heritage. It is a central belief in the Judeo–Christian tradition, as well as in Islam and other world religions, that individuals and societies are ultimately responsible to God. Individual judgment after death is an explicit teaching in many religions within the tradition. In one classical account, for example, an individual's eternal rewards or punishments are determined by his or her responsibility for choices over a lifetime, choices to seek and abide by God's will or choices to defy that will and live in sin.[3] The notion of original sin as depicted in the *Genesis* account of the fall of Adam and Eve represents the religious insight that human nature itself is flawed in some profound fashion, that it is prone to sin and to the irresponsible use of freedom.[4] In the face of this primordial failing, the Judeo–Christian tradition offers means of atonement so that individuals and societies can be redeemed before a benevolent God. Central to the various specific schemes for atonement is the act of acknowledging responsibility for sin and asking for forgiveness. Thus, the notion of responsibility plays an indispensable role in the Judeo–Christian worldview. Put in more frankly religious terms, it would be hard to reconstruct the meaning of the Judeo–Christian framework without the concept of sin, whether it take the expression of individual failing typical of modern Christians or of the collective failing of a people typical of ancient Hebrews.[5]

After Responsibility

For several reasons, this classical notion of responsibility has lost its prominent place for many Americans at the end of the twentieth century. American society is becoming increasingly secular and less shaped by explicitly Judeo–Christian themes. To the extent that the notion of responsibility arose and developed within that religious framework, increased secularization has meant a decline in the cultural sense of sin and responsibility.[6] Moreover, this process of secularization has meant more than simply stepping away from or forgetting the dominant religious tradition. Many intellectual movements in Europe and North America in the nineteenth and twentieth centuries were animated by a more or less conscious rebellion against main themes in the Judeo–Christian tradition.[7] Important strains of idealism, naturalism, positivism, existentialism, Marxism, and pragmatism share a general rejection of the supernatural and a specific rejection of the notion of responsibility to God. Instead, these intellectual movements tended to stress responsibility to others—the species, history, nation, science, class, and nature—or to oneself.

From the point of view of the religious tradition, these interpretations of responsibility inevitably weakened the notion on two counts. First, the "death of God" in the new versions of responsibility necessarily means the replacement of an absolute notion with one that is relative. The standards of assessing responsibility would then have to vary with respect to those to whom one is responsible as well as with the general contingencies of time, place, culture, and so on. Second, to the extent that modern notions of responsibility tend to center on responsibility to oneself—to be a creator of value, to actualize personal potential, to live a healthy lifestyle—they create the potential for the wholesale loss of standards. The reason for this lies in the paradoxical nature of the idea of responsibility to oneself.[8] Part of the general moral logic of responsibility is that one can be released from it by others to whom the responsibility is due. A home health care supervisor, for example, can release an occupational therapist from responsiblity for a specific aspect of a patient's therapy. A hospital risk manager may release a medical records professional from responsibility for a misplaced chart. A dentist owed payment for a procedure can free the patient of the obligation to pay. When this logic is applied to self-directed responsibility, the result is that the self is in a position to relieve itself of its own responsibilities. If I am responsible, for example, to live a healthy lifestyle and I realize that I am failing to do so, the "other" to whom I owe this responsibility is also myself. I can relieve myself of the general responsibility ("I really don't have to live a healthy lifestyle") or this particular expression of it ("I'll start my diet next week"). Whereas some selves (or consciences) set high standards and are demanding, even recriminating, other selves are permissive and accommodating. Therefore, if responsibility to the self is the primary or main responsibility, it has highly variable norms.

This philosophical conundrum takes on a more practical and culturally significant expression in twentieth-century psychology, which has helped to create "a therapeutic culture".[9] A central theme in this development is a tendency to regard the feeling of guilt, the typical emotional accompaniment of taking responsibility for one's failings, as pathological in itself. Many therapeutic techniques share the goal of identifying feelings of guilt and their sources and attempting to remove or weaken them by diffusing the sense of personal responsibility to which they are attached. For example, the feelings of guilt that may haunt an individual at middle age after a divorce may be seen through analysis to have originated in unreasonable expectations imposed by the parents of the divorced individual. This insight helps to resolve the guilt and allows the individual to move on and to "take responsibility" for the future without guilt for decisions made in the past and without feelings about them that were imposed by others. Plainly, this too brief moral analysis of twentieth-century psychoanalysis is unjust to the complexity of that phenomena and to its many good effects. Nonetheless, the role of psychoanalysis in the lessening of the contemporary sense of responsibility is too apparent to overlook.

Bureaucracy and Law

A second modern phenomena that has altered our sense of responsibility, especially personal responsibility, is the increasingly complex bureaucratic dimensions of contemporary life.[10] People must deal with large bureaucra-

cies in the workplace (both in their own employment and in the other businesses they deal with), in government, and even in the more private activities of love and marriage, recreation, communication, and entertainment. An
older world of individual artisans had already been replaced by assembly lines
and production teams by the middle of the twentieth century. The rise of the
service industry in the second half of the century has further increased the
complexity of working relationships as most services require highly articulated organizational structures. Even directly personal services like those provided by professionals in medicine, dentistry, and law, areas in which small
group or solo practice has been the norm, tend now to be organized into larger
associations or networks of providers and frequently into "chains."

One result of this interdependence and integration of contemporary life is
a spreading out and thinning of the notion of individual accountability. Rarely
is one individual personally and solely responsible for a decision, whether it
leads to success or failure. Even in the periodic exceptions to this general
tendency, when a single individual clearly has sole responsibility, there are
multiple opportunities for relocating and diffusing responsibility. The death
of a patient during surgery, for example, may appear at first to be the sole
responsibility of the anesthesiologist who administered the wrong sedative,
but an organization as complex as the surgery suite of a hospital has many
other layers of responsibility. Besides the anesthesiologist others on the surgery team attended the patient, and their timely intervention might have made
a difference. Perhaps some of these persons could and should have prevented
the death. Moreover, the hospital itself bears some responsibility for the institutional context that made such an accident possible. Was the system for
identifying and labeling sedatives properly designed and implemented? Was
it reviewed and updated regularly? Was the competency of the anesthesiologist assessed? There are also professional, state, and federal regulations—or
lack of them—that may have played some role in the patient's death. Yet once
it is admitted that the surgery team, the entire hospital, various accrediting
bodies, and the U.S. government all bear some responsibility, the classical
notion that a single individual is accountable for a bad outcome has been left
far behind.

Finally, the litigiousness of American society has also served to erode the
traditional notion of moral responsibility. This point is especially clear in the
area of medical malpractice. Often the most morally appropriate response by
a doctor after a medical mistake is to admit responsibility for the mistake and
apologize to the patient. Ironically, this may also be the course of action that
makes injured patients less likely to sue.[11] Yet admission of responsibility and
apology are just the wrong strategies in an environment in which lawsuits
against doctors have become so common and doctors' fear of them so pervasive. The obvious strategy for doctors who have made a mistake in such a
litigious environment is denial and the construction of defensive mechanisms

in anticipation of a potential lawsuit. In this adversarial environment, the simple, moral, and even religious act that promotes reconciliation ("I am responsible and I am sorry") has become a virtually impossible utterance for legal reasons.

These modern phenomena conspire against the classic notion of responsibility. A more complete account would have to acknowledge as well the important contributions each of these phenomena have made in sophisticating and curbing abuses in the main religious tradition. Frequently, the central themes of the Judeo–Christian tradition have been presented in a superficial and literally unbelievable fashion. Too often, false certitudes about divine standards of judgment have provided the basis for cruel and foolish human judgments. Modern psychology has fostered many important insights about the human condition, and psychotherapy has helped relieve many from excessive and self-defeating burdens of guilt. Many people have found renewal and a new sense of responsibility from such therapy. For all the negative consequences of bureaucracy, activities involving many interdependencies must have a social structure. Many aspects of contemporary bureaucracy are designed not only for efficiency, but also to encourage multiple contributions and shared decision-making. The committee meeting is one of the prices paid for a relatively democratic and open society. Medical malpractice law and litigation are important protections of patient rights and a method of compensation for real injuries. Evolution of the law in this regard has been an important partner in the establishment of respect for patient autonomy. Moreover, malpractice litigation is an expression of a genuine problem. Litigation would be unnecessary were there no medical malpractice. A more complete analysis of American culture would have to develop these and other positive aspects of these large-scale social phenomena.

Having admitted the incompleteness of this picture, however, it is important to note the role each of these has played in the lessening and even erosion of contemporary notions of responsibility. The stakes are high indeed. It is difficult to see how earnest commitment to the other values already articulated here, especially respect for dignity, service to the common good, and concern for the most vulnerable, is possible without a robust sense of responsibility. The dignity of the individual is the foundation for self-determination and for the right to informed consent in a clinical contexts. This idea of dignity could not operate practically without an assumption that providers and patients are responsible for their choices, at least for some choices and to some degree. The value of the common good would be empty without acknowledgment of responsibility toward it. The interests of the least well-off cannot be protected unless individuals assume responsibility for protecting them. Therefore, the notion of responsibility is critical to these and to other moral values. It must be defended conceptually and applied vigorously but sensitively.

Subsidiarity

One point of entry into the complexities of responsibility in the practical world of the health care system is through use of a principle rooted in the Judeo–Christian tradition, particularly in Catholic political philosophy, namely, subsidiarity.[12] This principle presumes multiple levels of responsibility between individual and collective choice and directs that responsibility be tied to the appropriate levels for accomplishment of the various tasks at hand. The general insight in the concept of subsidiarity is that responsibility for a task should not be assigned at a more complex or higher level of organization unless the task cannot be performed competently at any less complex or lower level of organization.

Application of the principle of subsidiarity begins with the responsibilities of the least complex level of organization, namely, the individual person, who is to be assigned responsibility for tasks within that person's natural competence. A competent adult would be assumed to be responsible for a wide range of activities, especially those concerned most directly with that individual's personal life. Many tasks, however, are beyond the competence of an individual, especially immature, frail, or disabled individuals. The next appropriate level of responsibility is the family. Families are the primary structures for creating social life and for the care of children, the elderly, and the sick or disabled. Yet many of the problems facing families are insuperable if left to families themselves. Therefore, higher levels of organization, such as neighborhood associations, churches, school districts, business, and local government, must be called on to perform tasks beyond the competence of families. Public health measures such as garbage collection, pest control, and immunization programs are plainly beyond the competence of families and therefore fall naturally to this next level.

Local organizations themselves are faced with tasks that require movement to the next stage. County services for drug and alcohol abuse, for example, may require assistance from a statewide system of financing and access to professionals. States in turn have their own responsibilities: operating the Medicaid program, regulating health insurance, and licensing and disciplining health care professions. Finally, some tasks are beyond the competence of states and can be performed competently only by the federal government. Medicare is the obvious example, the program through which the federal government provides financing and sets national norms for the health care of Americans over the age of sixty-five.

The principle of subsidiarity begins with a presumption in favor of the individual and of less complex and voluntary organizations and legitimates the employment of more complex organizations and government involvements only as they are necessary for the accomplishment of socially important tasks.

Viewed from the other direction, the principle also holds that if a task must be done, and it cannot be done at any lower level, then it must be assigned to a higher level of organization. The principle, therefore, is not hostile to "big government" when large-scale federal involvement is needed for the task at hand. It is hostile to "big government" only if government absorbs the proper responsibilities of lower levels of organization by assuming tasks that the states, the marketplace, or individuals could perform competently. Subsidiarity is a very flexible and contextual principle, tilting toward neither individualism nor any form of collectivism. Instead, it requires prudential determination of the social tasks that must be done and the proper place to assign the responsibility for doing them. Its starting place is the individual, and it always favors the less complex organization.

Although the principle of subsidiarity has explicit religious roots, it has a certain obviousness to Americans. The United States' political tradition of individual rights and federalism in the relationship between the national government and the states captures much the same insight.[13] The Bill of Rights articulates a political disposition in favor of the individual and therefore of individual initiative and responsibility for choices. The U.S. Constitution defines the tasks that must be performed by the federal government and reserves other powers for the states. States themselves have developed relationships with their own counties and municipal governments for the distribution of responsibility for tasks internal to the state. Therefore, the idea of distributing responsibility from individual through various forms of private association and local, state, and federal government is, on secular grounds, a familiar one to Americans.

Federal Lessons

Questions about what tasks are most naturally the responsibility of what level of organization are complex and situational and cannot be addressed adequately in general terms. Nonetheless, some lessons seem clear from the experience of health care delivery systems in the United States and around the world and from recent debates about systemic reform. To begin at the level of greatest complexity, it seems a fair generalization from American experience with Medicare and from other nations' health care systems that the federal government's most important role lies in determining a basic benefits package and in organizing some method of financing to ensure universal access to it.[14]

There are examples where the government has taken a direct hand in health care provision, in the United States' Veterans Administration system and in the United Kingdom, for example, but these seem the exceptions rather than the rule. More important, to do so appears to violate the main directive of the principle of subsidiarity. There are plainly less collective ways to provide health care, through the private and voluntary sectors, for example. In fact, recent history with the Medicare program suggests that the federal government may have already overstepped its natural province. For example, the role of HCFA (Medicare's Health Care Financing Administration) in shaping hospital admission and length of stay at the local level seems in principle to have stepped over other important levels of organization, namely, local or state initiatives.[15] On the other hand, it appears that there is no other entity of less complex organization than the federal government that could determine a basic benefit package for health care and ensure that it is made available to all Americans.

There can be legitimate debate, of course, as to whether these tasks must be done at all. Some hold, for example, that there should be no basic benefit package and no commitment to universal coverage.[16] However, arguments already made about human dignity and its link to a right to health care are incompatible with this position. Beginning, then, with the assumption that this is a task that must be accomplished, that there must be universal access to a basic benefit package, there appears to be no entity of less complexity than the federal government that can accomplish this necessary task. No doubt, there are many ways in which the federal government might discharge the responsibility for such a task. The principle of subsidiarity would be a helpful guide in helping to choose the best method or methods. For example, faced with a choice between a method of financing that is operated totally by a federal bureaucracy on lines similar to Social Security versus an arrangement in which the federal government regulates private health insurance companies or state health insurance plans, the principle of subsidiarity would suggest a choice of the latter, assuming, of course, that the job can be done equally well in either case. However, this is precisely where complex questions of efficiency and equity arise. In such areas, details make all the difference and general advice is of little use.

States' Duties

The role of the states in health care is also complex and cannot be determined in detail outside of context. Here again, however, recent history can be a useful guide in applying the insights of subsidiarity. Although it has served the needs of millions of Americans who would have had no other recourse, the Medicaid program is in many respects a disaster.[17] It is certainly a failure compared with its companion program, Medicare. This is clear in contemporary politics. Despite its problems, Medicare is defended vigorously by politicians. A politician who called for abolition of the program, for a change in eligibility, or for a substantial reduction in benefits would have a most difficult time being reelected. At the same time, Medicaid is a political orphan. Politicians are competing to restrict eligibility, to impose reductions in services and restrictions of choices in the program, and to reduce or eliminate federal involvements.

One of the reasons for the difficulties of the Medicaid program is the assignment of responsibility for determining program eligibility to the states. This has the immediate implication of creating not only a variety of circumstances for care for the poor around the United States (a circumstance not wrong in itself), but also a situation in which the poor in the poorer states (the poorest of the poor) fare worse than the poor in the wealthier states.[18] Individuals who are eligible for Medicaid in one state can be ineligible according to the criteria used in others. To appreciate the inequity this creates, imagine that Medicare covered everyone over age sixty-two in Wisconsin but only those over seventy-five in Arizona. The problem with variable norms will only increase as more Medicaid authority is passed to the states.

Therefore, as a general solution to underwriting the needed health care for those who cannot provide it for themselves, the Medicaid program approach of locating responsibility at the state level appears to have failed. The lesson here is that universal coverage should involve the wholesale transfer of this responsibility from the states to the federal government, either by eliminating the Medicaid program altogether in a scheme of universal insurance or by federalizing the Medicaid program so that, like Medicare, there is a single standard for eligibility and an equitable method of financing across the nation.

Networks

An important recent phenomena at a lower level of organization is the development of health care plans or networks that bring together providers and insurers into one organization, typically using some forms of capitated financing. The HMO is the prototype of this health care plan.[19] Application of the principle of subsidiarity applied here would stress the responsibility of the health plan for the immediate care of its enrollees subject to state and federal guidelines.

A deeper practical problem as these plans evolve within a competitive framework is assignment of responsibility for the health needs of the community. A health care plan that uses capitation and that is competing with other health care plans will naturally seek to enroll the healthiest members of the community because they use fewer resources from the health care plan. The logic of capitation (payment per member per month whether care is needed or not and little or no payment at the time of care) is clear financially: The less care provided, the better the financial health of the health care plan. This logic can lead to irresponsible choices concerning individuals. For financial reasons, enrollees might be denied needed specialty care or necessary hospitalization.[20] Perhaps these potential abuses can be avoided or minimized by rigorous quality control and by the evolution of detailed practice protocols.

It is plain that health care professionals have the immediate responsibility to ensure that they are providing the best care possible for the individuals that they serve. However, this simple imperative is made more complex in an environment in which health care networks have made cost containment an insistent value. Thus, one of the new responsibilities of professional groups is to develop and refine practice protocols, critical pathways, and other standards for providing care that balance the demands of quality with cost containment. Defining practice protocols is naturally the province of the professions because no one else is as competent to do it. However, subsidiarity might also demand that, having defined these parameters, professionals may not be competent to enforce them on themselves and certainly not on hospitals and health care networks. Although professionals may evolve these protocols, government, through courts, legislation, or regulation, may have to enforce them.

The negative social impact of competing capitated networks may be harder to contain. Members of the community who have higher than average health care costs will be avoided by all the competing health care plans.[21] Who is, or rather who should be, responsible for the high risks, the very sick, the poor who are sicker than average, and the overutilizers in any given community? If these persons cannot be cared for within the logic of the voluntary associations that make up competing health care plans, then subsidiarity demands that the state or federal government regulate these plans to ensure that the interests of the least well-off are served. In other words, the health care marketplace operating on its own principles may be incapable of accomplishing the necessary tasks of caring for the least well-off. If so, a higher level of organization is needed.

Families

Families are the least complex social organization beyond the individual. As health care is becoming less centralized in hospitals and more community based, families are being asked to do more for their sick and disabled members than ever before. It is also clearer than ever before that habits rooted in family life—of eating, drinking, working and recreation—have important effects on the overall health of individuals. Families therefore play an important role in prevention as well as in the care of their own members.

Yet while more is being asked of families, the nuclear family unit is at the same time under unprecedented pressure. There are many communities in the United States, for example, in which the vast majority of births are out of wedlock, and the vast majority of households are headed by a single parent. There are health implications associated with these phenomena.[22] Under these circumstances, it is hard to see how families can assume the new burdens expected of them from the health care delivery system. Unless these trends can be reversed and the family unit reinvigorated or unless the family is reinvented in a fashion that provides more mutual support for its members, the responsibilities that have been assigned primarily to families will have to be moved to another level of responsibility. In fact, this is already an obvious cultural phenomenon in the United States: functions typically provided in the past by families are being perfromed by social service agencies in the voluntary and governmental sectors. Whereas this arrangement may solve some practical problems, it creates others. In particular, it tends to depersonalize and bureaucratize human relationships.

Individual Determinism

The lowest level of social organization, of course, is the individual, and that is the point at which our secular and religious notions of responsibility most naturally rest. Here the forces that have been eroding the conception of responsibility become the clearest and the most troubling from the point of view of both health policy and clinical care. Are individuals responsible for the state of their own health? Or, to make the normative issue clearer, should individuals be held responsible for the state of their own health? Two opposing answers are possible here, each containing some validity.[23]

The first is a form of determinism that minimizes or rejects the role of personal responsibility. For the determinist, the more that is understood about genetics, the effects of early childhood education and experiences, the impact of socioeconomic status, and the natural and social environment itself, the more that is understood about the impact of these factors, the less room there is for personal responsibility. In addition to the obvious genetically inherited diseases, there is also evidence now that obesity, alcoholism, and perhaps even nicotine addition have a genetic component.[24] Although smoking cessation appears to be primarily an act of personal choice, patterns of cigarette smoking suggest that it is easier statistically to stop smoking (or not start) if an individual is a white woman with a college education compared, for example, with an African–American man who has less than a high school education.[25] Nobody chooses or merits their gender, race, and initial socioeconomic circumstances; so how much individual responsibility is involved in the choice to smoke cigarettes or to stop?

Moreover, particular comparative assessments of responsibility are exceptionally difficult to make. For example, how are personal responsibilities best assessed in cases in which a peer-conscious teenager begins to smoke cigarettes in practical ignorance of the health effects, only to find years latter, when the effects are clear, that it seems impossible to quit? How does this level of responsibility compare with someone who was never tempted to smoke cigarettes or who found the act of quitting relatively simple? It may long remain a mystery why some people are so immediately and strongly addicted to cigarette smoking and others are not, and why among the former group some succeed in ending their addiction and others try to end it constantly with little or no success. With the little that is known now, can we treat the cigarette smoker with emphysema differently than someone with emphysema unassociated with cigarette smoking? Can we hold the smokers who do not (cannot?) stop smoking personally responsible for the health implications of a personal habit?

When the traditional concept of responsibility is applied to these cases, there is a tendency to regard individual choice as *the* cause and to ignore the multiple layers of other causes that shaped this cause itself.[26] Focus is on the act of the alcohol abuser, the act of drug abuse, the act of high-risk sexual behavior; but in each of these cases and in all cases involving choices and habits that can be destructive of health, there are multiple causes going back again to genetics, psychology, and socioeconomic facts. People are inclined to judge, for example, that an individual lost his life to lung cancer *because* he smoked. Yet it may also be true that he would not have developed lung cancer had his parents not smoked, had he not been given free cigarettes in the military, had cigarette advertising been banned, had cigarettes been made safer, or had the government not subsidized tobacco. Although all these causes may have been necessary for the result, focus is often placed exclusively on the one cause believed to be most directly under the agent's immediate control.

Yet from the determinist perspective, it is arbitrary to elevate one cause above all others. Moreover, every cause, including the allegedly "free choice" to smoke, has causes, and those causes have causes, and so on. Personal responsibility then vanishes from this perspective. Moreover, elimination of responsibility is proper and beneficial because the notion of responsibility is often regarded by determinists as a placeholder for blaming. Because he smoked, he is responsible; therefore, he is to be blamed for his own death from cancer; but if the determinist perspective is correct, this amounts to blaming individuals already victimized by their circumstances. It makes as much sense on this account to blame a smoker who has lung cancer as it would to blame someone for having inherited cystic fibrosis or having contracted tuberculosis from a sneeze on the street. Victim-blaming has no place in the health care arena because by imputing guilt it increases the burden of suffering on those who are already sick. It also tends to undermine the natural sympathies of health care providers by fostering the view that some patients are unworthy of health care because their medical conditions are "their own faults."

Free Will

The other perspective, the free will position, is the more traditional. It insists on a decisive role for personal responsibility. Regardless of genetic inheritance, the impact of parents and early childhood, socioeconomic status, and so on, the phenomenon of choice is one of the most self-evident facts about human psychology. People are not responsible for everything that occurs in their lives, not even everything they do. Yet there are plainly times when individuals consider alternative actions and choose to do one thing and avoid another. Circumstances like genetic disposition, overbearing parents, unfortunate social and economic circumstances may mitigate responsibility in some cases but can never fully overwhelm it. Moreover, even when no choice is made, persons can be held responsible by virtue of what they should have chosen. People can be guilty of negligence.

From this point of view, the determinist alternative appears to regard human beings as robots, as simply playing out scripts developed by genes interacting with the environment. Determinism thus undermines the conception of human dignity and the very reasons that support respect for individual self-determination. It also seems false from an introspective point of view. People do experience the phenomena of voluntary choice: planning for the future, weighing present alternatives, releasing tension in an act of choice, "knowing" retrospectively that things could have been otherwise. Moreover, the fact that some people, despite their circumstances, do change their habits and do become more responsible in their choices indicates that it can be done.

Furthermore, the determinists' view that all action is caused is an artificial device for creating political categories of "voluntary victims," individuals who refuse personal responsibility and impute blame to others or to society as a whole.[27] It is not the child abuser's fault; the blame lies with his own abusive father. The crack addict who robs a convenience store is not responsible; it is society's fault. (This is a curious twist in the determinist position here, as blame of any sort is generally associated with free will and responsibility. If neither exists, can an abusive father or society be blamed any more than the agent in question?) Voluntary assumption of the role of victim operates as a personal and collective denial, a denial of freedom and responsibility. Yet this is a morally unstable denial because it is self-deceptive. People know that they are free, that they could have chosen other actions, other habits. Denial is, to use a phrase from philosopher John-Paul Sartre, a matter of "bad faith," a matter of knowing that there is an appropriate level of personal responsibility yet denying it to others and to oneself.[28]

Holding Two Views

These views tend to exclude one another. The first account holds that there is no personal responsibility; the second account holds that there is. This dispute is a metaphysical dilemma of primary importance.[29] For reasons already outlined, the free will perspective must be true, or at least people must act as if it is true in order for other values to be taken seriously. Nonetheless, the concerns of the determinist that this amounts merely to a strategy of blaming the victim, a worsening of already bad circumstances, and a hardening of caregivers' attitudes constitute an important practical limitation on the application of personal responsibility.

There is an intuitively plausible strategy for combining insights from both views. Health education and the development of policy must assume the traditional, common sense perspective that people are free, that they can be responsible. People can change bad habits into good ones and therefore are, to some extent, responsible for some parts of the state of their own health. This allows for educating, urging, praising, and blaming.

At the same time, however, it must be admitted that the ability to determine the degree of personal responsibility in any given case is theoretically and practically limited and that attempts to do so are fraught with negative personal and social consequences.[30] When holding a person responsible amounts to blaming the victim, this is a cruel and gratuitous addition to suffering. When health care professionals divide patients into the responsible and irresponsible, the deserving and undeserving, the good and the bad, sympathy is diminished. Therefore, when it comes to caring for people in need, the insight of the determinist should be controlling. Regardless of how a patient's emphysema was caused, the health care needs of those suffering from emphysema must be addressed by health care providers. At the same time that responsibility is encouraged through education about the perils of cigarette smoking, for example, there should be no moral judgments about those who suffer from its effects. They should be treated with sympathy as if they were simply victims of circumstances beyond their control.

A kind of stereoscopic social vision is required, one that will forever be in tension with itself theoretically: an assumption of free will and responsibility before the circumstances of need and an assumption of determinism in clinical contexts. A clear and robust concept of personal responsibility is needed, but there must also be safeguards against abuses. In the health care area, use of the concept of personal responsibility is essential, but it cannot be allowed to violate the first premise of medical ethics: First, do no harm.

Notes

1. Susan Sauve Meyer, *Aristotle on Moral Responsibility* (Oxford: Blackwell Publishers, 1993), 18.
2. Hans Jonas, *The Imperative of Responsibility* (Chicago: Chicago University Press, 1984), 92-72.
3. For the development of this view, see Everett Ferguson, editor, *Doctrines of Human Nature, Sin, and Salvation in the Early Church* (New York: Garland Press, 1993).
4. Dietrich Bonhoeffer, *Creation and Fall: a Theological Interpretation of Genesis 1-3*, trans. by John C. Fletcher (New York: Macmillan, 1959). Philosopher Jean-Paul Sartre provides a secular account of a similar "original fall", namely, the shame of being (and not being) an object in the world. Sartre, *Being and Nothingness*, p. 384.
5. David Smith, *With Willful Intent: A Theology of Sin* (Wheaton, Ill.: BridgePoint, 1993).
6. Karl Menninger, *Whatever Became of Sin?* (New York: Hawthorn Books, 1973).
7. See, e.g., Karl Lowith, *From Hegel to Nietzsche*, translated by David E. Green (Garden City, N.Y.: Doubleday, 1967); Patrick Gardner, ed., *Nineteenth Century Philosophy* (New York: Free Press, 1968); and Paul Kurtz, ed., *American Philosophy in the Twentieth Century* (New York: Macmillan, 1966).
8. See, e.g., Samuel Gorovitz, "Health as an Obligation," in *Encyclopedia of Bioethics*, ed. by Warren Reich (New York: The Free Press, 1978), 606-609.
9. Bellah et al., *Habits of the Heart*, pp. 134-138.
10. Peter Blau, *Bureaucrcy in Modern Society*, 3rd. edition (New York: Random House, 1987).
11. J. Fiesta, "Communication—the Value of an Apology," *Nursing Management* 25, no. 8 (1994): 14-16; and G. Lester and S. Smith, "Listening and Talking to Patients," *Western Journal of Medicine* 158, no. 3 (March 1993): 268-72.
12. Fred Kammer, *Doing Faithjustice* (New York: Paulist Press, 1991), 80.
13. William Riker, *The Development of American Federalism* (Boston: Kluwer Academic Publishers, 1987).
14. See, e.g., Emily Freidman, " Medicare and Medicaid at 25," *Hospitals* 64, no. 15 (1990), 38, 42, and 46.
15. L. Brown, "Political Evolution of Federal Health Care Regulation," pp. 17-37.
16. See, e.g., Robert Sade, "Medical Care as a Right: A Refutation," *The New England Journal of Medicine* 285 (December 2, 1971): 1288-92.
17. Generally, see John Iglehart, "Medicaid," *The New England Journal of Medicine* 328, no. 12 (1993): 896-900.
18. Bach et al., "Ethics and Medicaid: A New Look at an Old Problem," pp. 433- 41; and B. Goldman, "Can a Poor State Afford Not to Expand Medicaid," *Journal of Health Care for the Poor and Undeserved* 4, no. 3 (1993): 219-32.
19. Generally, see G. Povar and J. Moreno, "Hippocrates and the Health Maintenance

Organization: A Discussion of Ethical Issues," *Annals of Internal Medicine* 109, no. 5 (1988): 419-24.

20. See, e.g., C. Clancy and B. Hillner, " Physicians as Gatekeepers," *Archives of Internal Medicine* 29, no. 7 (1989): 84-85.

21. Eckholm, *New York Times*, p. 22.

22. K. Judge and M. Benzeval, "Health Inequities; New Concerns About the Children of Single Mothers," *British Medical Journal* 306, no. 6879 (1993): 677-80; and B. Compass and R. Williams, "Stress, Coping, and Adjustment in Mothers and Young Adolescents in Single- and Two-Parent Families," *American Journal of Community Psychology* 18, no. 4 (1990): 525-45.

23. Dougherty, "Bad Faith and Victim-Blaming," pp. 112-16.

24. L. Lumeng and D. Crabb, "Genetic Aspects and Risk Factors in Alcoholism and Alcoholic Liver Disease," *Gastroenterology* 107, no. 2 (1994) 572-8; R. Farell, "Obesity: Choosing Genetic Approaches from a Mixed Menu," *Human Biology* 65, no. 6 (1993): 967-75; and A. Heath and N. Martin, "Genetic Models for the Natural History of Smoking: Evidence for a Genetic Influence on Smoking Persistence," *Addictive Behavior* 18, no. 1 (1993): 19-34.

25. Aday, *At Risk in America*, pp. 75-80.

26. Dougherty, "Bad Faith and Victim-Blaming," p. 115.

27. Charles J. Sykes, *A Nation of Victims* (New York: St. Martin's Press, 1992).

28. Sartre, *Being and Nothingness*, pp. 86-116.

29. See, e.g., Sidney Hook, ed., *Determinism and Freedom* (New York: Collier Books, 1958).

30. Beauchamp and Childress, *The Principles of Biomedical Ethics*, pp. 358-60; and Dougherty, " Bad Faith and Victim-Blaming," pp. 112-16.

9

Excellence

Human Nature

The drive for excellence is a fundamental value. It is continuous with a phenomenon evident in the behavior of higher animals, namely, their apparent delight in the exercise of species capacities—flying, running, tracking prey, and so on. Similarly, humans delight in the exercise of their own specific capacities, taking pleasure in perfecting expressions of those capacities in art, science, communication, for example. Exactly which capacities are unique to humans is one of the most controverted questions in the history of thought. It amounts to the challenge of defining human nature.[1] Without diminishing the importance of all the subtleties that such a question entails and the range of opinions that have been put forth, there is a general framework for interpreting human experience that appears to recur though Western philosophy and theology.[2] Beginning as early as Plato, thinkers have identified a tripartite character in human nature.[3] Although these divisions are given varying names and their different aspects are stressed in many and sometime incompatible ways, expressed in the simplest terms, the three most important human capacities appear to be feeling, thinking, and choosing.

First, humans have the capacity to feel, including but going well beyond the biological capacities of experiencing pleasure and pain. Human feeling also includes the wealth of human emotional life, from the most mundane and familiar feelings of amusement, anger, and boredom, for instance, to the most abstract and episodic feelings associated, for example, with experiences of beauty, existential anxiety, and love for both real and hypothetical others. Virtually all human experiences have an emotional tone or coloration, and this is not infrequently their most important aspect.

Humans also have the capacity to think, which encompasses activities as diverse as composing a shopping list, making a business plan, and testing a scientific theory. Thinking, especially in practical contexts, frequently involves discovering or creating relationships between ends and means, between goals and ways of achieving them. Thinking also includes acts of insight into structure or content and contemplations of the meanings of things. It is also crucial in communication, allowing for the exchange of complex experiences through the medium of ideas and the words that express them.

Finally, humans have the capacity to choose. Again, this simple notion captures a diverse phenomenon, including quotidian choices that make and remake habits, defining moments of existential choice, and choices not to choose. Choices shape destinies in great and small ways. Often the most important thing that can be learned about a person is what he or she has chosen, does choose, and (probably) would choose.

Of course, these capacities interpenetrate each other in the unity of human experience. Feelings are woven throughout thinking and choosing. Thinking can reshape feelings and often issues in choice. Choices set the context for thinking and can expand and contract feelings. Yet each of these capacities has its own distinctive relationship to the drive for excellence. Feelings can be deepened, sensitivities widened and enriched. Thinking can become clearer and encompass more information and perspectives. Choice can become more generative and self-affirming. The drive for excellence itself, although it plainly has an emotional and rational dimension as well, seems most closely related to choice. It represents a choice to seek the ideal, to transcend the present, to struggle constantly to improve.

Foundations

Greek thinkers of the classical period, especially Aristotle, identified a connection between the drive for excellence and moral development.[4] The ancient Greek word for virtue, *arete*, meant being good at something.[5] The word in its original usage was incomplete. It had the sense of "being good at . . . " and suggested the question: Good at what? Politics, military matters, crafts?

It was the contribution of Greek philosophers to distinguish a kind of *arete* which meant good as a human being, excellence in being a person. The link to morality is that one of the special excellences available to humans is the integration of feeling, thinking, and choice into habits of behavior that constitute moral virtue. The virtue of courage, for example, represents the excellence of personality that integrates most appropriately the feelings aroused by danger, rational calculation of risks and alternatives, and a habit of choosing just the right response in changing situations.[6] The virtue of moderation is the excellence of personality that combines in the best manner attraction and resistance to pleasure, knowledge of the consequences of various indulgences, and a habit of selecting the right kinds and amounts of pleasure time after time.[7] Aristotle also held that the cultivation of such excellence in one's personality is, along with the contemplation of higher things and simple good luck, the chief ingredient of a happy life.[8] Virtuous people are generally happy people, not in the sense of giddiness and exhilaration, but in the sense of satisfaction and harmony. They have a sense of unity and wholeness, an integrity of personality that facilitates positive relationships with others and, most importantly, with themselves. In this sense, striving for moral excellence is its own reward. Excellence may well deserve reward, but it is not performed for the sake of reward outside itself.[9] Virtue is a component of a life that is most humanly satisfying because it seeks perfection in just those capacities that are distinctly human.

Because of its theology of sin and consequent need for redemption, the Judeo–Christian tradition has never been quite as sanguine about the link between virtue and happiness.[10] In most standard interpretations of the tradition, the cultivation of virtue is an obligation whether or not it is linked to the achievement of happiness. Simply put, seeking the personal perfection of moral virtue is a religious duty owed to God. Of course, in traditional theories of salvation, the link between virtue and happiness is reestablished supernaturally: Temporal virtue is rewarded with eternal happiness.

The general structure of striving for excellence is little changed by the addition of a religious framework, with one significant exception. Given the traditional Judeo–Christian belief in a personal and benevolent God, the drive for excellence is less a matter of creativity and human choice and more a matter of discerning one's divinely given talents and how their exercise can best advance the overall plan of creation. Therefore, the mechanisms for approaching excellence may appear the same on either a secular or religious account, but the latter provides a different and perhaps more insistent motivation. From a religious perspective, it is a matter of "getting it right."

This point cannot be pressed too far, however, because it is also clear that many individuals with no religious commitments have a consuming zeal for excellence, a sense of being driven toward an ideal. This is quite apparent in the arts and the professions but can be found in virtually every activity and walk of life. Performing well, regardless of how exalted or humble the task, is often linked closely to a person's self-esteem. It is a way of asserting one's distinctiveness through a defining superiority in some activity or characteristic. Being the best at something provides a rightful sense of pride, whether that best is confirmed by an award from a professional association or by being known as the best dentist in the community. At the same time that the secular world provides this natural support for the drive for excellence, a religious worldview can sometimes reverse the insistence of the drive. The confidence that comes from the belief that matters are ultimately under the control of a benevolent God can provide justification for an attitude akin to what William James called "moral holidays," a certain relaxed distancing from worldly standards of achievement.[11]

Corporate Excellence

The striving for excellence is not only an individual phenomenon but has social expressions as well. To the extent, often a great extent, that groups of people can share a self-identity, seeking excellence plays a role for groups similar to its role for individuals. A family, for example, can take pride in one of its members' achievements, not only as an individual accomplishment, but also as the work of the family unit. Neighborhoods, cities, and states tout their distinctive superiorities. Racial, ethnic, even gender pride as well as love of country can be expressions of an identification with the excellences of one's own group. This tendency, in fact, is such a strong natural disposition that it can easily become excessive and lead to dangerous corruptions. Egotism at the individual level, an excessive pride that is prejudicial to the interests of others, is reflected socially as racism, ethnic hatred, sexism, and the scourge of nationalism.

The social psychology of this phenomenon is complex but familiar. A strong sense of identification with a group—a loyalty—can unite deep divisions in the self. It can bring together, in Josiah Royce's phrase, "the inner and the outer," that is, that aspect of the self that seeks personal fulfillment in isolation and that part that wants satisfaction through involvement with society.[12] Close identification with the excellences and aspirations of a group can therefore be emotionally satisfying because it brings together personal fulfillment and social life. One is personally fulfilled in a social commitment. It is this emotional satisfaction in a corporate identity that produces some of the best and worst moral realities.

A structural similarity to the individual pursuit of excellence is clear in voluntary societies. Business corporations, for example, strive for excellence by trying to build organizational habits—a corporate culture—of striking a successful balance between the extremes of authoritarianism and anarchy in organization, stodginess and flamboyance in style, conformism and individualism in motivation, "hard" and "soft" in sales, etc.[13] What counts as the right balance varies with context. More anarchy can be expected in a small software company, less in a hospital; more stodginess in a law firm, less in a pediatrician's office; more conformism in an investment brokerage, less in a home health care agency; a "harder sell" at an automobile dealership, "softer" at a funeral home. Applying Aristotle's wisdom on behalf of commercial goals, businesses would be wise to assess the climate of expectations and the existing dispositions of their organizations and then seek excellence by "leaning against" these tendencies to seek greater balance.

They would also be wise to bind themselves to high standards, to commit themselves publicly to the pursuit of excellence.[14] This can be difficult for health care organizations at a time when survival in the face of frequent closures, downsizing, and "reengineering" can become an unspoken but dominant motive in an organization. In such an environment, excellence requires concerted efforts to provide mutual inspiration and support in pursuit of shared purposes. The alternative is mediocrity: "enforced conformity, timid nonaggressiveness based on mutual insecurity, losing sight of one's purpose, and retreating into suspicious collective self-protection."[15]

Quality

These general observations about excellence apply throughout the world of health care. Direct providers of care, administrators and payers, indeed persons throughout the health care system have individual drives toward excellence. Many institutions and corporate structures have explicit commitments to excellence in their field, sometimes with detailed goals and objectives. Those who are served by the health care system, both the insured and enrollees in health care plans as well as those who are served directly as patients, have expectations of excellence in health care contexts. The drive for excellence and the expectation of it in health care frequently take the expression of a commitment to quality.[16]

From the provider's point of view, the struggle to achieve and maintain high standards of quality in health care centers on three measures: outcomes, process, and patient satisfaction. The most obvious measure of the quality of health care is the health of the individuals and populations who are served. This is also the most objective of the three measures. When an antibiotic resolves an infection, when a cancer is removed by surgery, or when a pain is relieved, evidence of success is straightforward. When life expectancy is in-

creased in a community, when the infant mortality rate declines, or when more
cancers are detected at earlier stages, again quality is evident in outcomes.[17]

Yet even in this relatively objective arena, there are difficulties in determining excellence. Although the concepts of health and disease may be biological in their roots, they also have cultural, psychological, and contextual
dimensions that complicate measurement of success. While resolving an infection, for example, appears to be an unqualified success in its own right,
resolving an infection in a person who is terminally ill with metastatic cancer
may represent a merely technical excellence without sensitivity to the larger
context of quality of care. Removal of a cancer may also entail loss of a limb,
an organ, or a capacity. Pain is notoriously difficult to measure objectively; a
pain that drives one person to a doctor may be a pain that another accepts as
part of life.

Similar ambiguities bedevil assessment of the quality of health care across
populations. Life span may increase or decrease in a community because of
factors having nothing to do with health care efforts. For example, life span
generally rises when the overall level of education increases, and it generally
falls when levels of violence rise.[18] Infant morality rates may change as the
result of better nutrition, delayed parenthood, or changing rates of abortion.
Earlier detection of cancer is capable of enhancing quality only when effective treatments are available. In some cases, early detection of small, slow-
growing, nonthreatening cancers, some prostate cancers, for example, may
serve only to create anxiety or to provoke harm through unneeded interventions. In sum, individual and collective health outcomes are natural and frequently revealing indicators of excellence in health care, but they must be
used with circumspection.

Process measures can also help in attempts to assess the quality of care.[19]
Outcomes are often literally beyond the control of health care. Diseases can
worsen despite the best efforts of modern medicine, and of course patients
die. Even when everything is done properly, poor outcomes can result, sometimes because of the gravity of the condition and sometimes because of natural degenerative processes. At the same time, many medical conditions resolve
themselves without health care interventions because of the body's natural
inclination toward balance and its ability to heal. Other medical conditions
improve not because of health care interventions, but irrespective of them,
sometimes even in spite of them. Outcome measures alone, without supple-
mentation with assessment of quality in the processes of care, can thus be
profoundly misleading. The best regional oncology center, for example, may
have health outcomes far worse than a community hospital simply because
of the greater severity of illness in the population it serves. The best neonatal
intensive care unit in a city may have the highest rate of infant deaths simply

because its patients include large numbers of children whose mothers' received no prenatal care during pregnancy.

It is important, therefore, for professions and health care institutions to set and maintain process standards that are thought to be the best pathways to good outcomes even when good outcomes are not obtained. The challenge implied here is to combine the best of statistical reasoning—maintaining processes that are designed to achieve success overall in the long run—with the flexibility to respond to the unique demands of individual patients in the here and now. In other words, what is needed is consistency in providing good procedures without lapsing into "cookbook medicine."

Finally, there is the measurement of excellence from the point of view of those directly served.[20] As insured individuals, members of health plans, and taxpayers, consumers prize administrative efficiency and low cost in the health care system. Cost containment is the goal of the healthy. As patients, people have different goals. Then they want positive health outcomes and the best available processes. Access to quality care is the goal of the sick. Intangibles are also valued, including such diverse considerations as courtesy, a sense of being listened to, and emotional support through crises. Much of what is included under the caring aspect of health care is pertinent here. Patients may get the best medical outcome with the use of the best available processes and still feel that they were treated in an uncaring fashion. Of course, patient satisfaction can also be affected by less morally significant features, such as the affability of health care providers, amenities, and ease of parking; but it is unlikely that even a full range of these less significant items can substantially improve patient satisfaction with a health care encounter perceived to be uncaring in the moral sense. Excellence in health care therefore means not only the best processes and the best possible outcomes, but also high standards in caring for patients.

Provider Choices

Excellence, as noted above, is closely associated with choice. Therefore, another important dimension of ensuring quality in health care is guaranteeing an appropriate range of choice for both providers and patients. Provider choice begins with selection of a profession. Generally, quality is served when individuals perform functions they are best suited for and enjoy. A wide range of individual choice of health professions helps to maximize the likelihood of this result. Other important choices follow when health care professionals determine an area of specialization within their professions, including the choice of general practice. The challenges of a nursing career in public health, for example, are considerably different from those faced by a neonatal intensive care nurse. Similarly, there is a great difference between medical practice in pathology and family practice, between general dentistry and oral surgery, between pharmacy in a retail outlet or in hospital practice. Again, achieving "the best fit" between a person's talents and the demands of a specific occupation is generally best attained by assuring the widest range of individual choice.

On the other hand, however, provider choice must be balanced with attention to the demands of the marketplace and the needs of society. For example, many more nurses may prefer working in hospitals than the marketplace can support as hospitals contract and hospital care is replaced by community-based care. At the start of their careers, many more doctors may prefer to work in subspecialties than the nation needs, and far too few may prefer the primary care fields that are presently understaffed.[21]

The marketplace provides some of the incentives necessary to make the necessary adjustments: Job opportunities and salaries can erode where there is an excess of professionals and expand where there is a shortage. However, in some cases, steps by government to influence or regulate these choices are appropriate.[22] There are considerable public subsidies throughout the health care sector in general and in the education of health care professionals in particular. This investment provides a general moral justification for managing the supply of health professionals in light of the needs of society. In addition, the presence of insurance, barriers to effective comparison shopping, and the urgency of many health care needs make large parts of the health care sector immune to the normal workings of the "laws" of supply and demand. In many instances, an oversupply of hospital beds and doctors does just the opposite of what these economic laws predict: It drives prices up.[23] Even when market forces are effective, they can be unacceptably slow. Without strong government incentives and regulations, for example, it could take an intolerable length of time before the marketplace alone produces enough primary care doctors for the nation's needs. Considerable political prudence is required to manage the numbers of health professionals well, but some of the tools to do so are obvious, including expanding or restricting medical residencies, loan forgiveness and tuition support programs, enhancing or reducing reimbursement rates in Medicare and Medicaid, and adjusting licensure and the scope of practice laws.

Another important dimension of provider choice, especially in medicine, is connected to the spread of integrated delivery networks that bring together group practices of doctors, hospitals, and third-party payers. The dominant style of medical practice at mid-century, an individual doctor operating a solo practice, has been largely swept aside by the development of larger group practices. Now these group practices are being integrated into delivery networks, often by way of the employment of doctors by the networks. Financial arrangements have also moved rapidly from fee-for-service to capitation. These changes have contracted provider choice. Market pressures have forced doctors to accommodate themselves to these new realities, altering control over decision-making, styles of practice, and the financial dimensions of careers.

Given the rapidity and wholesale character of these changes, it might be important for providers and for the general public to create some competing incentives or regulations to ensure that independent practice and fee-for-service arrangements remain a viable option, at least for some doctors. For all their flaws, the moral challenges of the these older styles of practice are well known and therefore may be more manageable. Moving the health care system entirely away from these known models in a very brief time may overwhelm society's ability to assess and control the morally sensitive dimensions of the doctor–patient relationship. For example, if virtually all doctors become employees, the traditional moral consensus that discharge of fiduciary responsibility entails the freedom (and duty) to refer patients to the best provider for each patient's needs could easily be lost. This consensus is being eroded already by the rush to configure networks.[24] Despite the moral problem created (and some legal problems as well), the plain expectation at the sale of a doctor's practice to a network is that the doctor will refer his or her patients to—and only to—other network providers.[25] According to the traditional model, this is a frank conflict of interest; but if the whole medical profession is absorbed into competing delivery networks, a new moral consensus will have to be created and the same moral value, protection of patients, will have to be preserved in some other fashion.

Patient Choices

From the perspective of patients, choice of provider is exceptionally important. Much of health care, despite its technical dimension, remains a highly personal activity. The fit of personality between a doctor and a patient can be an important dimension of patient satisfaction, and thus of the quality of care. Moveover, this fit between doctor and patient is an important ingredient in developing and maintaining trust. How much choice is necessary in this respect is a matter of prudence. The goal of finding the ideal doctor for each patient is plainly unreasonable, but it is important that patients be able to avoid doctors with whom they are uncomfortable. The wide freedom of choice that many (insured) patients have enjoyed in the past is receding rapidly.[26] Employers are offering fewer insurance options, and more of these involve exclusive contracts with hospitals and with closed panels of doctors, that is, with HMOs in which the choice of hospital and doctor is limited. This contraction of choice will likely continue. Even in the worst case, however, significant choice could be preserved in a system in which patients are assigned a primary health care doctor, so long as patients have a negative choice, that is, the right to select another doctor if the first relationship proves unsatisfactory.

In determining the proper scope for consumer choice of doctors, it is important to remember that in other areas of personal health care services, in nursing or physical therapy, for example, there is generally only this sort of negative choice. Typically, a nurse or physical therapist is assigned to a patient. Patients work with that professional unless they cannot or will not do so. That the situation regarding choice of doctors has been different historically is not a definitive argument that it must remain so. The nurse–physical therapist model may well become the dominant one for doctors in managed-care networks. The central ethical issue is to determine how much patient choice is needed to create and maintain an atmosphere of trust, a key ingredient in achieving excellence in health care.

Another difficult dimension of patient choice bearing on excellence involves biomedical research. This activity and its resulting technology have come to characterize American health care in the latter twentieth century. This has not been an unmixed blessing. Research and development of new drugs, surgeries, medical devices, and diagnostic instruments are costly enterprises. In some cases, they have been pursued inappropriately. They can create a sense of the impersonal and can fragment care by the subspecialization and bureaucracy they sometimes foster. Yet research and biomedical technology are certainly part of the excellence of contemporary health care, significant contributors to the dramatically expanded power to cure and to care that is the special achievement of this century. Fostering the best of this success while limiting its costs and abuses is one of the main challenges of health policy. At the center of the challenge is charting a new course for the modern academic health center. These centers are the research, teaching, and service sites in the vanguard of innovation in research and biomedical technology development; but pressures in local markets to cut hospital costs are rapidly making them economic dinosaurs.

Competition

A different strategy for maintaining high standards of quality throughout the health care system involves building and maintaining competition among providers. As a general economic strategy, competition can enhance quality by providing a range of consumer choice,[27] which will allow consumers to select the best affordable quality and, in effect, to drive poor and overpriced services from the marketplace.

Competition works best under certain conditions: when producers can move easily in or out of a field of economic activity, when consumers have some discretion about whether and when to buy, and when consumers can readily compare both quality and price. Much of health care is ill-suited to competition because these conditions do not prevail.[28] First, it is most difficult for providers to move in and out of health care activities. Key health professions require long years of education and clinical training. Moreover, most direct providers of care are members of professions that are guaranteed a monopoly of practice through state licensing laws. Many delivery organizations in health care, like hospitals, visiting nurses associations, and dental practices, are especially difficult to open and close. Second, the insistent character of many health care problems allows little discretion on the part of patients or burdens patient use of discretion with the risk of a worsened medical condition. Moreover, patients do not purchase most of their health care directly; a doctor's order is needed. Finally, it is exceptionally difficult for even the most intelligent and dedicated consumer to compare the quality of care among doctors, hospitals, and other professional and institutional providers. There are simply too limited reliable comparative data available.

The value of competition, therefore, is more limited in health care than in other areas of the economy. Nonetheless, some degree of competition is still useful to preserve choices for both providers and patients and to help maintain pressures for high quality and low prices. The current public policy question is not whether competition is appropriate in health care, but rather what kinds of competition are appropriate and what are the proper moral limits of competition. As a general rule, those limits are reached when the health care provider–patient relationship is undermined, the health care needs of communities are not addressed, or the destructive consequences of competition outweigh its benefits. In too many contemporary contexts, the moral limits of health care competition have been reached or exceeded.

Quality of Life

A final important dimension of excellence in the health care arena involves troubled issues related to quality of life. Access to needed health care is only one aspect of the general quality of life, which also includes relationships with family and friends, work environment, education, arts and entertainment, and physical environment. When used in a health care context, however, "quality of life" typically refers to the independence and capacities that can be diminished or lost when health care is successful *only* in maintaining life it-self or life in an exceptionally compromised state. Cases that have raised the most controversy involve patients who have been trapped in the twilight state of irreversible coma or who linger with debilitating conditions and dementia in nursing homes. Under such conditions, some would hold that quality of life is gone or reduced to an unacceptable level. There is biological life in these conditions, to be sure, and each moment of life increases its quantity. Miss-ing, however, are all or most of the excellences that biological life typically supports for human beings.

There are two extreme positions regarding the validity of the use of qual-ity of life assessments when it comes to making practical clinical decisions about patient care.[29] On the one hand is the position that might be called *vitalism*, which regards human life as a value in and of itself, something that is intrinsically worthy irrespective of any and all compromise or diminishment in its condition. From this perspective, talk of quality of life is dangerous not only because of its inherent subjectivity and potential for discrimination against those with handicaps, but also because of the general disrespect for the value of life that it may encourage. The primary goal of medicine in this viewpoint is the preservation of life. This view is often held for religious reasons, life being regarded as a gift from God, who alone may determine the time and circumstances of death. There are also secular grounds for holding this view. It is, for example, against the law to kill a person regardless of diminished quality of life. This prohibition creates an important legal standard of behav-ior and provides protection against arbitrary or discriminatory taking of life.

At the other extreme is a position that can be characterized as *nihilist* with respect to the intrinsic value of human life. It holds that human life itself has no intrinsic value. Human life is valuable only to the extent that it supports other activities that have intrinsic value, for example, self-awareness, com-munication, and independence. People holding this general view differ among themselves on the proper practical significance it should have in the care of terminally ill patients and those with very compromised quality of life. Many support physician-assisted suicide or euthanasia of those whose quality of life is radically diminished, absent, or soon-to-be absent.[30] In this viewpoint, the direct taking of a human life raises no troubling ethical questions because, in principle, life is without value. Others may support liberalizing doctor-assisted suicide laws but not euthanasia, as the former entails the active involvement and (presumably) voluntary participation of the patient, whereas the latter suggests the "mercy killing" of those who are incompetent. Still others may hold this view about life and still oppose physician-assisted suicide and eu-thanasia on practical grounds. One could hold, for example, that biological life alone has no value for humans, but that the potential abuses of allowing people to take life directly, even involving persons in such diminished states, would be far worse than the benefits created by more permissive suicide and euthanasia laws. As a rule, however, people holding this general nihilistic view are skeptical of the value of aggressive medical care when some level of quality cannot be sustained.

There is a middle ground that can negotiate between these extremes, a moral balance. It holds that human life does have an intrinsic value regardless of its quality, but that in some severely diminished states of quality, medical means to sustain life can properly be withheld or withdrawn. In this view, diminished quality of life never justifies killing or assisting in killing, but it can justify allowing an individual to die even when medical means exist to prolong life. In cases of terminal illness, medical interventions should be used with the sole purpose of maximizing comfort and easing the dying process, targeting the goal of achieving the "least worst death" for every patient.[31] This could take the form of hospice or hospice-like (that is, aggressive) pain relief, psychosocial support, and palliative treatment of medical conditions.

This middle ground is consistent with the main thrust of the Judeo–Christian tradition.[32] There is a deep reverence for life in the tradition (in spite of well-known and numerous failures to express this reverence practically) that makes the nihilist position untenable. A believer in the tradition simply cannot hold that life itself can become wholly without value, but it is also difficult within the tradition to accept an unqualified vitalism. How, for example, can one account for the behavior of martyrs and other heroes within the tradition who gave or risked their lives for other important religious or moral values? These numerous examples teach the message that the ultimate purpose of human life is spiritual, not biological. From this perspective, desperate struggles for increased quantity of life when quality sufficient to support life's spiritual goals are gone appears unbelieving, even idolatrous. Generally, human biology supports and sustains the spiritual, but in some diminished conditions when this is no longer true, human biological life has reached whatever potential it is capable of. Then choices can be made in favor of other values.

This moderate position is also at the heart of the distinction between ordinary and extraordinary measures, distinguishing, respectively, between procedures that must be provided and accepted for moral reasons and those that are futile or overly burdensome and can therefore properly be refused, withheld, or withdrawn.[33] This conceptual resource within the dominant religious tradition allows for *acceptance* of death under certain conditions. However, with certain exceptions (e.g., self-defense and just warfare), the mainstream of the tradition opposes killing and suicide. The key distinction here is between allowing to die and killing. The latter (killing) is rejected but not the former (accepting death). In fact, on this religious account, acceptance of an inevitable and proximate death as the apparent will of God is itself thought to be a form of excellence, even one of life's highest.

Balance

It is worth recalling, in conclusion, another bit of advice from the Greece of the classical period. Excellence, whether moral or physical, is to be obtained by striking the right balance between opposing tendencies. Excellence, according to Aristotle, is determined by a "golden mean" that finds just the right balance between two extremes.[34] Courage, for example, is that habit of choice that falls midway between a cowardice that collapses before the emotional repulsion to danger and a recklessness incapable of rational calculation of risk. Finding such a mean is not a mathematical exercise, not literally an exercise of averaging. Instead, it involves the cultivation of a refined intuitive sense, rather like the development of personal tactfulness, scientific "hunching," or the artistic sense that somehow knows that any more would be too much but any less too little.

Identification of the path to excellence is also highly contextual. Just as the same amount of medication can be too much for a small person and too little for a large person, so assessment of the golden mean must appraise differences of situation and personality. Aristotle advised an initial diagnosis of existing imbalances in one's personality and in the situation. Virtue was to be sought by systematically choosing the path closer to the other extreme than that toward which personality and situation predisposes. Timid persons develop courage, for example, by choosing actions they might otherwise regard as a bit too reckless. Rash persons excel by developing habits of choosing actions they might otherwise regard as overly cautious. Just as a crooked pipe is straightened by applying pressure against the direction that it bends, against its curve, so excellence is achieved by leaning against unbalanced dispositions.

There is an important lesson here for assessment of the health care system, its institutions, professionals, consumers, and patients, that is, for all of us. Cultivation of excellence and the maintenance of high quality require an honest diagnosis of existing extremes in emotional reactions, patterns of thinking, and habits of choice. Then there must be a resolve to reform, to turn back to reform, by leaning against these extremes in the design of institutions and the behavior of individuals.

Notes

1. Peter Langford, *Modern Philosophies of Human Nature* (Boston: Kluwer Academic Press, 1986); and Peter Carruthers, *Human Knowledge and Human Nature* (New York: Oxford University Press, 1992).
2. See, e.g., Francis Fukuyama, *The End of History and the Last Man* (New York: Avon Books, 1992), 143-98.

3. Plato, *Republic*, 676-88.
4. W.K. Guthrie, *The Greek Philosophers* (New York: Harper and Row, 1975).
5. Ibid., p. 8.
6. Aristotle, *Nichomachean Ethics*, pp. 71-79.
7. Ibid., pp. 79-85.
8. Ibid., pp. 14-23.
9. Robert C. Solomon, *Ethics and Excellence* (New York: Oxford University Press, 1992), 157.
10. See, e.g., Frederick Copleston, *A History of Philosophy, Vol. 2, Medieval Philosophy, Part II* (New York: Image Books, 1962), pp. 118-31.
11. William James, *Essays in Pragmatism*, ed. Aulburey Castell (New York: Hafner Press, 1948), 155.
12. John K. Roth, ed., *The Philosophy of Josiah Royce* (Indianapolis, Ind.: Hackett Publishing Co., 1982), 273-88.
13. See, e.g., Graig Hickman, *Creating Excellence: Managing Corporate Culture, Strategy, and Change in the New Age* (New York: New American Library, 1984); and John Kotter, *Corporate Culture and Performance* (New York: Free Press, 1992).
14. Tom Peters, *In Search of Excellence* (New York: Harper and Row, 1982).
15. Solomon, *Ethics and Excellence*, p. 157.
16. L. Wyszewianski, "Quality of Care: Past Achievements and Future Challenges," *Inquiry* 25, no. 1 (1988): 13-22.
17. L. Tancredi and R. Bovbjerg, "Creating Outcomes-based Systems for Quality and Malpractice Reform," *Milbank Quarterly* 70, no. 1 (1992): 183-216.
18. On the link of lifespan to social factors, see E. Rogot, P. Sorlie, N. Johnson, "Life Expectancy by Employment Status, Income, and Education in the National Longitudinal Mortality Study," *Public Health Reports* 107, no. 4 (1992): 457-61.
19. R. Coffey et al., "An Introduction to Critical Pathways," *Quality Management in Health Care* 1, no. 1 (1992): 45-54.
20. P. Cleary and B. McNeil, "Patient Satisfaction as an Indicator of Quality Care," *Inquiry* 25, no. 1 (1988): 25-36.
21. P. Burdetti, "Achieving a Uniform Federal Primary Care Policy," *JAMA*, 269, no. 4 (1993): 498-501.
22. For both sides of this issue, see J. Hawkins, "Should the Government Further Regulate Physician Supply? No." *Hospital Health Network* 67, no. 17 (1993): 10; and D. Satcher, "Should the Government Further Regulate Physician Supply? Yes." *Hospital Health Network* 67, no. 17 (1993): 10.
23. Eli Ginzberg, "The Grand Illusion of Competition in Health Care," *JAMA*, 249, no. 14 (1983): 1857-59.
24. American Hospital Association, *Toward Community Care Networks* (Chicago: AHA, 1993).
25. Generally, see D. Vavala, "Medical Practices: Hot Properties of the 90s," *Physician Executive*, 19, no. 5 (1993): 40-45.
26. Eckholm, *New York Times*, p. 22.
27. Dougherty, *American Health Care*, pp. 135-147.
28. Dougherty, *American Health Care*, pp. 135-147.
29. Richard McCormick, "To Save or Let Die," *JAMA* 229, no. 2 (1974): 172-76.
30. See, e.g., Howard Brody, "Assisted Death: A Compassionate Response to a Medi-

cal Failure," *The New England Journal of Medicine* 327, no. 19 (1992): 1384-88; and Timothy Quill, Christine Cassel, and Diane Meier, "Care of the Hopelessly Ill: Proposed Guidelines for Physician-Assisted Suicide," *The New England Journal of Medicine* 327, no. 19 (1992): 1380-84. For the other side of the debate, see George Annas, "Death by Prescription," *The New England Journal of Medicine* 331, no. 18 (1994): 1240-43; and Edmund Pelligrino, "Compassion Needs Reason Too," *JAMA* 270, no. 7 (1993): 874-75.

31. Margaret Battin, "The Least Worst Death," *Hastings Center Report* 13, no. 2 (1983): 13-16.
32. McCormick, "To Save or Let Die," pp. 172-76.
33. Beauchamp and Childress, pp. 200-202.
34. Aristotle, *Nichomachean Ethics*, pp. 44-52.

10

Conclusion

Problems

In spite of the collapse of recent systemic reform efforts, government is still pursuing incremental reforms at several levels.[1] Some employers have been mandated to make insurance available (but not to pay for it). Voluntary insurance-purchasing alliances have been formed. Other improvements in health insurance and the delivery system are still being crafted. The real energy for change, however, is now in the marketplace, where the American health care system is in a period of rapid transition, a period of fundamental "rationalization" and "re-engineering." Provider networks are expanding. Alliances and mergers abound. Hospitals are downsizing and closing as in-patient care is moved to new sites. Managed care and capitation are ascendant. Doctors, hospitals, and insurers are forming new partnerships, making doctors employees in unprecedented numbers.

These changes raise special challenges in the areas of access, cost control, and quality. Tens of millions of Americans are uninsured and will remain so into the foreseeable future. Lack of insurance creates significant barriers to care and frustrates efforts to improve health status. Fear of the loss of insurance though pre-existing illness exclusions creates job immobility and keeps some away from needed care. Access problems remain acute in America's inner cities and in large parts of rural America. The kind of access many Americans receive is dictated by the system's continuing predilection for acute-care services. Prevention, primary care, and long-term care remain areas of significant under-service. Moreover, market changes are exacerbating these access problems. Recent declarations that the provision of health insurance to employees is not an obligation of business, especially not small business, will probably lead more businesses to reduce or eliminate employee coverage. New competitive pressures on providers make commitment to uncompensated care for the uninsured less attractive than before—and far more dangerous economically.

Despite numerous efforts, cost escalation remains a significant problem as well. Health care continues to absorb an increasingly large portion of the nation's GDP and as a result threatens the general health of the economy. Rising costs have stressed business and household budgets. Attempts to address cost problems through downsizing, competition, and increased regulation of clinical contexts have raised concerns about quality. These changes have undermined morale among health care professionals, especially among doctors. Continued scrutiny is necessary to ensure that dissatisfaction resulting from these pressures does not erode standards of care.

In general terms, there is tension between the three goals of assuring universal access, controlling costs, and ensuring high quality. Viewed abstractly, their relationships seem locked in a "zero-sum" game: Progress in one area means losses in one or both of the other two. Assuring access for more people, for example, seems to entail new costs, diminished quality, or both. Containing costs appears to mean serving fewer people, serving them less adequately, or both. Maintaining high quality means paying more directly, paying indirectly by reductions in access, or both.

Nevertheless, the practical successes of other nations in Europe, Asia, North America, and Australia and of Medicare, despite its problems, indicate that nations can provide a basic package of care for all of their citizens at a reasonable cost and can do so with standards of quality that their citizens accept. The challenge facing those who want genuine reform in the United States is to fashion a plan or plans for the interaction of these goals that will reflect American experiences and the nation's best moral values.

Values

Values are states of affairs taken to be intrinsically desirable. Their ideal nature regulates behavior through attraction. An important subset of values in general are moral values. These values are ubiquitous in human experience. They may be well defined, but as a rule they tend to be vague. Rarely conscious, they are implicit throughout human activity. Moral values spring spontaneously to the fore, even in situations in which little or no conscious effort has been made to involve them. Values can be richly emotional, accounting for the passion and bitterness that often accompany value disputes. Moral values are practical in the sense that they guide behavior. Finally, moral values are deep, giving activities and life itself a sense of direction and purpose.

Values are taught to children at early ages and reinforced by culture in general. They are carried by a nation's traditions, especially its religious traditions. In the United States, the dominant religious tradition that has shaped moral values is the Judeo–Christian tradition. The American reflection of the European Enlightenment has also provided an important secular source of moral values. There are, of course, numerous alternative sources of moral values. Increasing numbers of Americans identify with other religious traditions or with none at all. Some do not identify with the Enlightenment tradition, or at least not with some key elements of it. Moral values can therefore be disparate and thus can lead to significant conflict.

An historically significant strategy for dealing with diversity in moral values is appeal to the metavalue of toleration, allowing maximal individual freedom to hold and act on differing values. As important as it is in many contexts, the strategy of toleration is ineffective in some disputes, especially those involving intolerance. The tradition of toleration has also helped to foster some trends that can be subversive of moral values themselves, particularly those that produce moral relativism, nihilism, and excessive individualism.

Despite these challenges, the practical character of health care guarantees that some moral values will be used to direct and control change in the system, whether they are used self-consciously or not. If there is to be reform, a genuinely better health care system must emerge from these changes. One mark of reform is a better fit between the health care system and Americans' most important moral values, which in spite of increased diversity, remain linked to the Judeo–Christian and Enlightenment traditions.

Dignity

One of the most significant moral values shaping American experience, respect for persons, is grounded in a conception of human dignity. The concept of dignity entails that each individual has a special, incalculably great value, a value to be distinguished in principle from the price of things. One source of the concept of individual dignity is religious. Most specific religions within the Judeo–Christian framework ground the idea of the special worth of each individual in the individual's spiritual destiny and relationship to God. The most significant secular source of the same value is the European Enlight-

enment and its American expression in commitment to explicit and enforce-
able individual rights.

Respect for individual human dignity in the health care arena has given rise
to the doctrine of informed consent, which protects the self-determination
of patients by ensuring that they are voluntary participants in their own health
care. Patients have the right to information about medical conditions and
available treatments and the right to refuse some treatments or to decline
health care altogether. Another important consequence of commitment to
human dignity is the claim of a right to a basic package of health care services for all persons. This claim provides the moral framework for insistence
on universal coverage. It also provokes the inevitable issues of defining a basic
benefit package and determining a means of delivering and financing it for all
Americans. These issues are special challenges in a libertarian climate of deep
distrust of government and commitment to an exaggerated form of individual
freedom.

Caring

The moral value of caring is at the heart of the project of health care. The
impulse to care is a response to human need and the special suffering that is
characteristic of many medical conditions. One dimension of caring is compassion, the ability of health care providers to "feel with" the pains and sufferings of their patients. Another key aspect of caring is fiduciary responsibility, the obligation of professionals to put the interests of their patients first in
any potential conflicts of interest and to avoid the creation of conflicts of
interests when possible.

Many pressures in the contemporary health care system, especially the trend
to treat health care like a business, threaten to undermine the ability of health
care professionals to keep the *care* in health care. They also threaten to create new and systematic conflicts of interest by pitting the financial interests
of providers against the medical interests of patients. Even the successes of
the informed-consent revolution has a shadow side in this arena. The new
adult-to-adult doctor–patient relationship is more open to a *quid pro quo*
understanding that can heighten the financial aspects of medicine to the detri-
ment of professional caring.

The Least Well-off

Protection of the least well-off is a moral value and serving their health care
needs a consequent moral imperative. This value and its obligations have

explicit biblical roots but can also be grounded in a secular sense of justice. Many Americans, especially those who are poor, less educated, and members of racial and ethnic minorities, have been underserved by the health care system and bear disproportionate burdens of morbidity and mortality. Moreover, as the health care system changes, especially as it changes under market pressures, these groups (as well as children, the frail elderly, and those with long-term mental and physical disabilities) are less able than others to assert their own interests in the process. The role of special-interest money and lobbyists in the defeat of the Clinton plan demonstrated that wealthy and powerful interest groups will have their say and will find ways to protect their most important interests. Less well-off Americans will have to rely on others to advocate for them.

Barriers to effective realization of this moral value include the increased coarseness and selfishness in national life and the marked tendency to devolve into "two Americas": a successful, optimistic, largely white majority versus a defeated, alienated, nonwhite minority. Establishing universal access to health care would go a long way toward realizing the value of protecting the least well-off, but more than universal coverage is necessary. Members of these groups require more than equal treatment to compensate for the health status disadvantages they have experienced historically and that they continue to experience.

The Common Good

Another barrier to caring for the least well-off is the general problem of caring for others in a society with a strong disposition toward excessive individualism. Balance demands that the moral value of respect for the dignity of each individual person be yoked to the moral value of service to the common good. Persons are inherently social, deriving much of what makes them individuals from their social environment and relationships with others.

The American health care system itself has deep social roots. It is based on clinical practice, experimentation, and science that has been accumulated and shared over generations. The system has benefitted in particular from important public investments in the second half of the twentieth century, especially in the construction of hospitals, education of doctors, and funding of care for the elderly. There are also important utilitarian and social contract considerations that make the case for more attention to the good of the whole. The moral value of service to the common good also underscores the need for greater emphasis on public health and preventive measures and for more opportunities for public input into decisions that shape the evolution of the health care system.

Cost Containment

The need to contain costs is not only an economic imperative, but also an important moral value. Waste is offensive economically but also wrong morally. Investing too many resources in health care can create unacceptably high opportunity costs as well as the harms caused by overtreatment. Responding to the demands of cost containment while expanding access and maintaining quality can be done only by grappling explicitly with the need to ration health care.

Rationing occurs now in the system and must be a feature of any system of health care distribution. The inevitability of adopting more explicit forms of rationing presents an opportunity for application of conscious ethical criteria. The need for specific forms of rationing must be demonstrated because of the potential for harms to persons and because of the possibility of violating the duty of easy rescue. Rationing should be done in the context of universal coverage for basic care and should be arranged so it will serve the common good and protect the most vulnerable. Important intangibles of caring and trust must be guarded carefully. Rationing must be based on an open process of priority setting, and it must avoid invidious discrimination. Finally, and most importantly, the Golden Rule insight must be observed: Those who ration should be subject to rationing.

Responsibility

Important issues surround the moral value of responsibility. There is a common-sense moral intuition that freedom and rights, indeed, any sense of personal or social authority, entails responsibility. There are obvious religious roots for this intuition in the Judeo–Christian tradition, the belief in a final judgment before God representing the ultimate form of accountability. Yet many trends in contemporary American society tend to undermine a robust sense of responsibility: an increasing disposition to regard moral agents as victims, the pressures of large bureaucracies, and the marked litigiousness throughout society. A renewed sense of moral responsibility can be anchored by the concept of subsidiarity, which directs that responsibilities follow the logic of appropriate assignment of tasks. Responsibility begins with individuals and moves to larger organizations only as lesser ones are unable to perform tasks that must be accomplished. Therefore, the best government is the least government *necessary to performing its appropriate tasks.*

Acknowledging the importance of responsibility means grappling with the difficult metaphysical problem of freedom versus determinism. There is a sense in which causes and events beyond individuals' control do determine the fates of individuals. This is especially clear in some health care arenas, genetics, for example. Yet there is another perspective from which individuals must be presumed to be free and encouraged to assume wider responsibilities for their lives and states of health. There is no easy resolution to this conceptual tension, but in health care it is prudent to emphasize freedom and responsibility in the areas of health education, prevention, and policy development and to adopt a more deterministic view of individuals in clinical contexts. Persons are free when they are urged to stop smoking, determined when they suffer from lung cancer, regardless of the cause.

Excellence

The drive for excellence is an important moral value. In one sense it lies at the very heart of the notion of valuing itself. Both values and the drive for excellence are orientations toward ideal states. There appears to be a natural human desire to use and perfect the most basic human skills so that sensitivity is expanded, reasoning becomes more comprehensive, and choices are made more adequate. This occurs in social organizations as well as within individuals. The drive for excellence in health care is frequently centered on the notion of quality. Although an inevitably evasive concept, quality can be measured in part by improved medical outcomes, by uniform use of appropriate procedures in the delivery of services, and by increased consumer satisfaction. A considerable range of choice by providers and patients is a precondition for setting and maintaining high standards of quality.

Quality as a form of general excellence is also involved in the concept of quality of life as a criterion for making health care decisions, especially for the dying. In such contexts, a spectrum of positions can be identified: from a vitalism that holds that all human life, regardless of quality, has inherent value, to a form of nihilism that denies value to human life below some level of quality. Interpreted not as a judgment about the value of life but as a way to assess the reasonableness of medical interventions, quality of life judgments can be useful for striking a balance between these extreme positions. Attaining balance is itself a form of excellence closely identified with the achievement of virtue. It represents a classical "golden mean" that can help provide prospective on the appropriate role of health care in the general quest for excellence in human living.

Making *Good* Time

These moral values may not be the only important ones at stake in the changing health care system. Perhaps those that are considered here have not been examined adequately. A task of this nature requires a self-consciousness of the possibility of omission, error, and even offense to others whose deeply held moral values are ignored, slighted, or misconstrued.

Yet these risks must be accepted for three reasons. First, they follow from the nature of the task. If values are as vague and open-ended as characterized here, then explicit articulation of them will necessarily be incomplete and approximation the best that can be expected. Second, this account is offered as a moment in a larger national conversation about who we are as a people and what can be expected from health care and the health care system. The reader is invited to reply, to correct, to reject, and thereby to contribute to making the conversation more complete. Most books are written alone; certainly this one has been. All books, especially this one, are nonetheless social acts drawing on the thoughts and achievements of others and inviting dialogue indefinitely into the future.

Finally, these risks are accepted because of the conviction that this project is of fundamental importance. As the health care system continues to change— rapidly and in fundamental ways—it is a certainty that medical, economic, political, and legal concerns will have important roles in determining the health care system of the future. It is less certain that moral values will be given their proper weight, however. Only if they are can there be any grounds for confidence that a changed health care system will be a reformed health care system, a system better in terms of the things most important to most of us.

This work began with an anecdote about an airplane without direction making "great time." That plane is the health care system; market changes the storm tossing the plane where it will and without direction, but direction must be provided if health care change is to amount to a better system, to health care reform. Moral values are the directional equipment that can point us back to reform. If this can be done, a genuinely better health care system may still emerge. Then making great time can also mean making good time, *morally* good time.

Notes

1. Jane White, ERISA May Hinder States As They Attempt Healthcare Reform," *Hospital Progress* 75, no. 8 (1994): 14-16; Marilyn Moon and John Holahan, "Can States Take the Lead in Health Care Reform? *JAMA* 268, no. 12 (1992): 1588-94; and John Iglehart, "Health Care Reform: The States," *The New England Journal of Medicine* 330, no. 1 (1994): 75-79.

Bibliography

Aday, Lu Ann, *At Risk in America* (San Francisco: Jossey-Bass, 1993).
———, James House, Karl Landis, and Debra Umberson, "Social Relationships and Health," *Science*, 241 (July 29, 1988): 540-545.
Agich, George, "Medicine as Business and Profession," *Theoretical Medicine*, 11, no. 4 (Dec. 1990): 311-324.
Altman, Lawrence and Elisabeth Rosenthal, "Changes in Medicine Bring Pain to Healing Profession," *New York Times* (February 18, 1990): 1 and 20.
American Hospital Association, *Toward Community Care Networks*, (Chicago: AHA, 1993).
Annas, George, "Death by Prescription," *The New England Journal of Medicine*, 331, no. 18 (Nov. 3, 1994): 1240-1243.
Aristotle, *Nichomachean Ethics*, trans. by Terence Irwin (Indianapolis, Ind.: Hackett Publishing Co., 1985).
Attfield, R., *A Theory of Value and Obligation* (London: Croom Held Ltd., 1987).
Axinn, June and Mark Stern, *Dependency and Poverty: Old Problems in a New World* (Lexington, Mass.: Lexington Books, 1988).
Bach, Marilyn, Charles Oberg, Nicholas Bryant, and Jeri Boleman, "Ethics and Medicaid: A New Look at an Old Problem," *Journal of Health Care for the Poor and Underserv*ed, 2, no. 4 (Spring 1992).
Barber, J., "Telling the Public the Real Health Cost Story," *Hospitals*, 66, no. 12 (June 20, 1990): 68.
Battin, Margaret, "The Least Worst Death," *Hastings Center Report*, 13, no. 2 (April 1983): 3-6.
Beauchamp, Tom and James Childress, *The Principles of Biomedical Ethics*, 4th edition (New York: Oxford University Press, 1994).
Beauchamp, Tom and Ruth R. Faden, "The Right to Health and the Right to Health Care," *Journal of Medicine and Philosophy*, 4, (1979): 119-131.
Bellah, Robert, Richard Madsen, William Sullivan, Ann Swidler, and Steven Tipton, *Habits of the Heart* (Berkeley, California: University of California Press, 1985).
Bevis, E., "Alliance for Destiny: Education and Practice," *Nursing Management*, 24, no. 4 (April 1993): 56-61.
Blackwell, B., "A Piece of My Mind; No Margin, No Mission," *JAMA*, 271, no. 19 (May 18, 1994): 1466.
Blau, Peter, *Bureaucracy in Modern Society*, 3rd. edition (New York: Random House, 1987).
Blendon, Robert, Mollyann Brodie, and John Benson, "What Should Be Done Now That National Health System Reform is Dead?" *JAMA*, 273, no. 3 (January 18, 1995): 243-244.

————, Mollyann Brodie, Tracy Hyams, and J. M. Benson, "The American Public and the Critical Choices for Health Care Reform," *JAMA*, 271, no. 19 (May 18, 1994): 1539-1544.

————, and Karen Donelan, "The Public and the Emerging Debate Over National Health Insurance," *The New England Journal of Medicine*, vol. 232, no. 3 (July 19, 1990): 208-212.

————, Karen Donelan, Graig Hill, Ann Scheck, Woody Carter, Dennis Beatrice, and Drew Altman, "Medicaid Beneficiaries and Health Reform," *Health Affairs*, vol. 12, no. 1 (Spring 1993): 132-143.

————, Andrew Kohut, John Benson, Karen Donelan, Carol Bowman, "Health System Reform: Physicians' View on Critical Issues," *JAMA*, vol. 272, no. 19 (November 16, 1994): 1546-1550.

————, John Martilla, John M. Benson, Matthew C. Shelter, Francis J. Connolly, and Tom Kiley, "The Beliefs and Values Shaping Today's Health Reform Debate," *Health Affairs*, vol. 13, no. 1 (Spring 1994): 274-284.

Blocker, Gene and Elizabeth H. Smith, *John Rawls' Theory of Justice* (Athens, Ohio: Ohio University Press, 1980).

Bok, Sissela, *Lying* (New York: Vintage Books, 1979).

Bonhoeffer, Dietrich, *Creation and Fall: a Theological Interpretation of Genesis 1-3*, translated by John C. Fletcher (New York: Macmillan, 1959).

Brody, Howard, "Assisted Death: A Compassionate Response to a Medical Failure," *The New England Journal of Medicine*, 327, no. 19 (Nov. 5, 1992): 1384-1388.

Brown, L., "Political Evolution of Federal Health Care Regulation," *Health Affairs*, 11, no. 4 (Winter 1992): 17-37.

Burdetti, "Achieving a Uniform Federal Primary Care Policy: Opportunities Presented by National Health Reform," *JAMA*, 269, no. 4 (Jan. 27, 1993): 498-501.

Burner, Sally, Daniel Waldo, and David McKusick, "National Health Expenditures Projections Through 2030," *Health Care Financing Review*, 14, no. 1 (Fall 1992): 1-30.

Butler, S., "A Tax Reform Strategy to Deal with the Uninsured," *JAMA*, 265, no. 19 (May 15, 1991): 2541-4.

Califano, Joseph A., "'The Challenge to the Health Care System: Can the Third Biggest Business Take Care of the Medically Indigent?' A Personal Perspective," *Health Care for the Poor and Elderly: Meeting the Challenge*, ed. Duncan Yaggy (Durham, N.C.: Duke University Press, 1984).

Callahan, Daniel, "Reforming the Health Care System for Children and the Elderly to Balance Cure and Care," *Academic Medicine*, 67, no. 4 (April 1992): 219-222.

————, *Setting Limits* (New York: Simon and Schuster, 1987).

Caplan, Arthur, Daniel Callahan, and Janet Hass, "Ethical and Policy Issues in Rehabilitation Medicine," *Hastings Center Report*, Special Supplement (August 1987): 1-20.

Carmody, John, *Ecology and Religion: Toward a New Christian Theology of Nature* (New York: Paulist Press, 1983).

Carr, David, *Educating the Virtues: An Essay on the Philosophical Psychology of Moral Development and Education* (New York: Routledge, 1991).

Carruthers, Peter, *Human Knowledge and Human Nature* (New York: Oxford University Press, 1992).

Cassirer, Ernst, *The Philosophy of the Enlightenment*, trans. By Fritz Koelln and James Pettegrove (Boston: Beacon Press, 1955).

Chelimsky, Eleanor, "The Political Debate About Health Care: Are We Losing Sight of Quality?" *Science*, 262 (Oct. 22, 1993): 525-528.

Christensen, S., "The Subsidy Provided Under Medicare to Current Enrollees," *Journal of Health Politics, Policy, and Law*, 17, no. 2 (Summer 1992); 255-64.

Churchill, Larry, *Rationing Health Care in America* (Notre Dame, Indiana: University of Notre Dame Press, 1987).

———, *Self Interest and Universal Health Care* (Cambridge, Mass.: Harvard University Press, 1994).

Clancy, C. and B. Hillner, "Physicians as Gatekeepers," *Archives of Internal Medicine*, 29, no. 7 (July 1989): 84-5.

Cleary, P. and B. McNeil, "Patient Satisfaction as an Indicator of Quality Care," *Inquiry*, 25, no. 1, (Spring 1988): 25-36.

Coffey, R., J. Richards, C. Remmert, S. LeRoy, R. Schoville, and P. Baldwin, "An Introduction to Critical Pathways," *Quality Management in Health Care*, 1, no. 1 (Fall 1992): 45-54.

Collins, James, *The Thomistic Philosophy of Angels* (Washington, D.C.: Catholic University Press, 1947) .

Committee for the Study of the Future of Public Health, *The Future of Public Health* (Washington, D.C.: National Academy Press, 1988).

Compass, B. and R. Williams, "Stress, Coping, and Adjustment in Mothers and Young Adolescents in Single- and Two-Parent Families," *American Journal of Community Psychology*, 18, no. 4 (Aug. 1990): 525-45.

Copleston, Frederick, *A History of Philosophy, Vol. 2, Medieval Philosophy, Part II* (New York: Image Books, 1962).

Cotton, P., "Preexisting Conditions 'Hold Americans Hostage' to Employers and Insurance," *JAMA*, 265, no 19 (May 15, 1991): 2451-3.

Dailey, J., H. Teter, and R. Cowley, "Trauma Center Closures: a National Assessment," *Journal of Trauma*, 33, no. 4 (Fall 1992): 539-46.

Daniels, Norman, *Am I My Parents' Keeper?* (New York: Oxford University Press, 1988).

Deckard, M. Meterko, D. Field, "Physician Burnout: An Examination of Personal, Professional, and Organizational Relationships," *Medical Care*, 32, no. 7 (July 1994): 745-54.

Dolenc, Danielle A. and Charles J. Dougherty, "DRGs: The Counterrevolution in Financing Health Care," *Hastings Center Report*, 15, no. 3 (June 1995): 19-29.

Dougherty, Charles J., *American Health Care: Realities, Rights, and Reforms* (New York: Oxford University Press, 1988).

———, "Bad Faith and Victim-Blaming: The Limits of Health Promotion," *Health Care Analysis*, 1, no. 3., (1993): 111-119.

———, "Ethical Dimensions of Healthcare Rationing," (St. Louis, Catholic Health Association, 1994).

———, "Ethical Values at Stake in Health Care Reform," *JAMA*, 268, no. 17 (Nov. 1992): 2409-12.

———, "Equality and Inequality in American Health Care," in *Freedom and Equality*, ed. Esther MacKintosh (Washington, D.C.: Federation of State Humanities Councils, 1992).

———, "Joined in Life and Death: On Separating the Lakeberg Twins," *Bioethics Forum*, vol. 11, no. 1 (Spring 1995): 9-16.

——, "The Common Good, Terminal Illness, and Euthanasia," *Issues in Law and Medicine*, 9, no. 2 (Fall, 1993): 151-166.

——, "The Costs of Commercial Medicine," *Theoretical Medicine*, 11 (1990): 275-286.

——, "The Excessess of Individualism," *Health Progress*, 73, no. 1 (Jan. 1992): 22-28.

——, "Values in Rehabilitation: Happiness, Freedom, and Fairness," *Journal of Rehabilitation* (January/February/March 1991): 7-12.

——, and Sandra L. Dougherty, "Moral Reconstruction in the Hospital: A Legal and Philosophical Perspective on Patient Rights," *Creighton Law Review*, 14, no. 4, supplement (1980-1981): 1409-1434.

Dyer, Allen, "Ethics, Advertising, and the Definition of a Profession," *Journal of Medical Ethics*, (11 June 1985): 72-78.

Eckholm, Erick, "While Congress Remains Silent, Health Care Transforms Itself," *The New York Times* (Dec. 18, 1994): 1 and 22.

Emmanuel, L., "Advance Directives: What Have We Learned So Far?" *Journal of Clinical Ethics*, 4, no. 1, (Spring 1993): 8-16.

Engelhardt, Tristram, "Why a Two-tier System of Health Care Delivery is Morally Unavoidable," in *Rationing America's Medical Care: The Oregon Plan and Beyond*, ed. by Martin Strosberg, Joshua Weiner, Robert Backer, and Allen Fein (Washington, D.C.: Brookings Institution, 1992), 196-207.

Ezzy, D , "Unemployment and Mental Health: A Critical Review," *Social Science and Medicine*, 37, no. 1 (July 1993): 41-52.

Faden, Ruth R. and Tom L. Beauchamp, *A History and Theory of Informed Consent* (New York: Oxford University Press, 1986).

Farell, R., "Obesity: Choosing Genetic Approaches from a Mixed Menu," *Human Biology*, 65, no. 6 (Dec. 1993): 967-75.

Feinberg, Joel, "The Nature and Value of Rights," *Rights, Justice and the Bounds of Liberty* (Princeton, N.J.: Princeton University Press, 1980).

Ferguson, Everett, editor, *Doctrines of Human Nature, Sin, and Salvation in the Early Church* (New York: Garland Press, 1993).

Fiesta, J., "Communication—the Value of an Apology," *Nursing Management*, 25, no. 8 (Aug. 1994): 14-6.

Fishkin, James, *Democracy and Deliberation: New Directions for Democratic Reform* (New Haven, Conn.: Yale University Press, 1991).

Franks, Peter, Carolyn M. Clancy, and Martha R. Gold, "Health Insurance and Mortality," *JAMA*, 270, no. 6 (Aug. 11, 1993): 737-741.

——, Paul A. Nutting, and Carolyn Clancy, "Health Care Reform, Primary Care, and the Need for Research," *JAMA*, 270, no. 12 (Sept. 22, 1993): 1449-1453.

Friedman, E., M. Hagland, T. Hudson, and P. McNamara, "The Sagging Safety Net: Emergency Departments on the Brink of Crisis," *Hospitals*, 66, no. 4 (Feb. 20, 1992): 26-40.

Freidman, Emily, "Medicare and Medicaid at 25," *Hospitals*, 64, no. 15, (Aug. 1990).

Fried, Charles, *Right and Wrong* (Cambridge, Mass.: Harvard University Press, 1978).

Fukuyama, Francis, *The End of History and the Last Man* (New York: Avon Books, 1992).

Gardner, Patrick, editor, *Nineteenth Century Philosophy* (New York: Free Press, 1968).

Gavaghan, H., "Genetics Business Booming Yet Uncertain," *Nature*, 369, no. 6478 (May 26, 1994): 341-2.

Ginsberg, Eli, "The Grand Illusion of Competition in Health Care," *JAMA*, 249, no. 14 (April 8, 1983): 1857–1859.

——, "Health Care and The Economy—A Conflict of Interests?" *The New England Journal of Medicine*, 326, no. 1 (Jan. 2, 1992): 72–74.

——, *The Road to Reform*, (New York: The Free Press, 1994).

Glaser, William, "The United States Needs a Health System Like Other Countries," *JAMA*, 270, No. 8 (August 25, 1993): 980–984.

Goldman, B., "Can A Poor State Afford Not to Expand Medicaid," *Journal of Health Care for the Poor and Underserved*, 4, no. 3 (1993): 219–32.

Goodin, Robert E., *Protecting the Vulnerable* (Chicago: University of Chicago Press, 1985).

Gorovitz, Samuel, "Health as an Obligation," in *Encyclopedia of Bioethics*, ed. By Warren Reich (New York: The Free Press, 1978).

Gustafson, James A., *A Sense of the Divine: The Natural Environment from a Theocentric Perspective* (Cleveland, Ohio: Pilgrim Press, 1994).

Guthrie, W. K., *The Greek Philosophers* (New York: Harper, 1975).

Hadley, Jack, Earl Steinberg, and Judith Feder, "Comparison of Uninsured and Privately Insured Hospital Patients," *JAMA*, 265, No. 3 (Jan. 16, 1991): 374–379.

Hadley, James P., "Overview," *Health Care Financing Review*, 15, no. 1 (Fall 1993): 1–5.

Harrington, Charlene, Christine Cassel, Carroll L. Estes, Steffie Woolhandler, David Himmelstein, and the Working Group on Long-Term Care Program Design, Physicians for a National Health Program, "A National Long-term Care Program for the United States," *JAMA*, 266, no. 21 (Dec. 4, 1991): 3023–3029.

Harris, Fred R. and Roger W. Wilkins, editors, *Quiet Riots: Race and Poverty in the United States* (New York: Pantheon Books, 1988).

Hart, H. L. A., *Law, Liberty, and Morality*, (Stanford, California: Stanford University Press, 1963).

Hawkins, J., "Should the Government Further Regulate Physician Supply? No." *Hospital Health Network*, 67, no. 17 (Sept. 5, 1993): 10.

Heath, A. and N. Martin, "Genetic Models for the Natural History of Smoking: Evidence for a Genetic Influence on Smoking Persistence," *Addictive Behavior*, 18, no. 1 (Jan 1993): 19–34.

Held, Virginia, *Feminist Morality* (Chicago: University of Chicago Press, 1993).

Hickman, Graig, *Creating Excellence: Managing Corporate Culture, Strategy, and Change in the New Age* (New York: New American Library, 1984).

Higgs, Robert, *Crisis and Leviathan: Critical Episodes in the Growth of American Government* (New York: Oxford University Press, 1978).

Hobbes, Thomas, *Leviathan*, ed. by C.B. Macpherson (Baltimore: Penguin, 1976).

Hook, Sidney, ed., *Determination and Freedom* (New York: Collier Books, 1958).

Hope, Marjorie and James Young, *The Faces of Homelessness* (Lexington, Mass.: Lexington Books, 1990).

Howe, Irving, editor, *1984 Revisited: Totalarianism in Our Century* (New York: Harper and Row, 1983).

Iglehart, John K., "Health Care Reform and Graduate Medical Education, "*The New England Journal of Medicine*, 330, no. 16 (April 21, 1994): 1167–71.

——, "Health Care Reform: The States," *The New England Journal of Medicine*, 330, no. 1 (Jan. 6, 1994): 75–79.

——, "Medicaid," *The New England Journal of Medicine*, 328, no. 12, (March 25, 1993): 896–900.

————, "Medicare," *The New England Journal of Medicine*, 327, no. 20 (Nov. 12, 1992): 1467–1472.

James, William, *Essays in Pragmatism*, ed. by Alburey Castell (New York: Hafner Press, 1948).

Jefferson, Thomas, *The Political Writings of Thomas Jefferson*, ed. by Edward Dumbauld (Indianapolis, Ind.: Bobbs-Merrill, 1955).

Jegen, Evelyn, and Bruno Manno, editors, *The Earth is the Lord's: Essays on Stewardship* (New York: Paulist Press, 1978).

Jenker, Nancy S. and Robert A. Pearlman, "Medical Futility: Who Decides?" *Archives for Internal Medicine*, 152 (June 1992): 1140–1144.

Jennings, Bruce, "A Grassroots Movement in Bioethics," *Hastings Center Report*, 18, no. 3 (June 1988): Supplement 1–16.

Jonas, J., S. Etzel, and B. Barzansky, "Educational Programs in US Medical Schools, 1993–94," *JAMA*, 272, no. 9 (Sept. 1994): 694–701.

Jonas, Hans, *The Imperative of Responsibility* (Chicago: Chicago University Press, 1984).

Joy, Donald, editor, *Moral Development Foundations: Judeo-Christian Alternatives to Piaget and Kohlberg*.

Judge, J. and M. Benzeval, "Health Inequities; New Concerns About the Children and Single Mothers," *British Medical Journal*, 306, no. 6879 (March 13, 1993): 677–80.

Kammer, Fred, *Doing Faithjustice* (New York: Paulist Press, 1991).

Kant, Immanuel, *Grounding for the Metaphyscis of Morals*, trans. by James W. Ellington (Indianapolis, Ind.: Hackett Publishing Co., 1981).

Katzner, Louis, "The Original Position and the Veil of Ignorance," in Blocker, Gene and Elizabeth Smith, editors, *John Rawls' Theory of Justice*, (Athens, Ohio: Ohio University Press, 1980): 42–70.

Kekes, John, *The Morality of Pluralism* (Princeton, N.J.: Princeton University Press, 1993).

Kendall, David and Will Marshall, "Health Reform, Meet Tax Reform," *The American Prospect*, Spring 1995: 74–78.

Kerrey, Bob and Philip Hofschire, "Hidden Problems in Current Health-Care Financing and Potential Changes," *American Psychologist*, 48, no. 3 (March 1993): 261–264.

Kleinman, L., J. Kosecoff, R. Dubois, and R. Brook, "The Medical Appropriateness of Tympanostomy Tubes Proposed for Children Younger than 16 Years in the United States," *JAMA*, 271, no. 16 (April 27, 1994): 1250–5.

Kotter, John, *Corporate Culture and Performance* (New York: Free Press, 1992).

Kurtz, Paul, editor, *American Philosophy in the Twentieth Century* (New York: Macmillan, 1966).

Langford, Peter, *Modern Philosophies of Human Nature* (Boston: Kluwer Academic Press, 1986).

Lawson, Bill E., *The Underclass Question* (Philadelphia: Temple University Press, 1992).

Leininger, M. ed., *Caring: An Essential Need* (Thorofare, N.J. Charles Stack, 1981).

Leopold, M., "The Commercialization of Biotechnolgy," *Annals of the New York Academy of Science*, 700 (Dec. 21, 1993): 214–31.

Lessnoff, Michael, *Social Contract* (Atlantic Highlands, N.J.: Humanities Press International, 1986).

Lester, G., and S. Smith, "Listening and Talking to Patients," *Western Journal of Medicine*, 158, no. 3 (March 1993): 268-72.

Lieberman, Jethro, *The Litigious Society* (New York: Basic Books, 1981).

Long, Stephen and M. Susan Marquis, "The Uninsured 'Access Gap' and the Cost of Universal Coverage," *Health Affairs*, vol. 13, no. 2, (Spring II, 1994): 211-220.

Lowith, Karl, *From Hegel to Nietzsche*, translated by David E. Green (Garden City, New York: Doubleday, 1967).

Ludden, J., "Doctors as Employees," *Health Management Quarterly*, 15, no. 1 (1st Quarter 1993): 7-11.

Lumeng, L. and D. Crabb, "Genetic Aspects and Risk Factors in Alcoholism and Alcoholic Liver Disease," *Gastroenterology*, 107, no. 2, (Aug. 1994) 572-8.

Lyons, David, *Rights* (Belmont, California: Wadsworth Publishing Company, 1979).

Maier, Paul, *First Christians: Pentecost and the Spread of Christianity* (New York: Harper and Row, 1976).

Marcel, Gabriel, *The Existential Background of Human Dignity*, (Cambridge, Mass.: Harvard University Press, 1963).

Maritain, Jacques, *Man and the State* (Chicago: University of Chicago Press, 1956).

Martin, Mike, *Self-Deception and Morality* (Lawrence, Kansas: University Press of Kansas, 1986).

McClellan, M. and R. Brooks, "Appropriateness of Care: A Comparison of Global and Outcome Methods to Set Standards," *Medical Care*, 30, no. 7 (July 1992): 565-86.

McCormick, Richard, "To Save or Let Die," *JAMA*, 229, no. 2 (July 8, 1974): 172-6.

McCoy, Timothy, "Biomedical Process Patents: Should They be Restricted by Ethical Limitations?" *Journal of Legal Medicine*, 13, no. 4 (Dec. 1992): 501-519.

McKay, N. and J. Coventry, "Rural Hospital Closures," *Medical Care*, 31, no. 2 (Feb. 1993): 130-40.

Mead, George Herbert, *Mind, Self, and Society*, ed. by Charles Morris (Chicago: University of Chicago Press, 1965).

Mehuron, Tamar Ann, editor, *Points of Light: New Approaches to Ending Welfare Dependency* (Washington, D.C.: Ethics and Public Policy Center, 1991).

Meiland, Jack and Michael Krauz, editors, *Relativism, Cognitive and Moral* (Notre Dame, Ind.: University of Notre Dame Press, 1982).

Menninger, Karl, *Whatever Became of Sin?* (New York: Hawthorn Books, 1973).

Meyer, Susan Sauve, *Aristotle on Moral Responsibility* (Oxford: Blackwell Publishers, 1993).

Mill, John Stuart, *On Liberty*, ed. by David Spitz (New York: Norton, 1975).

———, *Utilitarianism*, ed. by Samuel Gorovitz (Indianapolis, Ind.: Bobbs-Merrill, 1971).

Miltmann, Jurgen, *On Human Dignity: Political Theology and Ethics*, trans. by Douglas Meeks (Philadelphia: Fortress Press, 1984).

Moon, Marilyn and John Holahan, "Can States Take the Lead in Health Care Reform?", *JAMA*, 268, no. 12 (Sept. 23, 1992): 1588-1594.

Morris, J., D. Cook and A. Shaper, "Loss of Employment and Mortality," *British Medical Journal*, 308, no. 6937 (April 30, 1994): 1135-9.

Murray, Robert, *The Cosmic Covenant: Biblical Themes of Justice, Peace, and the Integrity of Creation*, (London: Sheed and Ward, 1992).

Nagel, Thomas, *The Possibility of Altruism* (Oxford: Clarendon Press, 1970).

Nelson, Lawrence, Westley Clark, Robert Goldman, and Jean Schore, "Taking the Train to a World of Strangers: Health Care Marketing and Ethics," *Hastings Center Report*, 19, no. 4 (Sept. 1989): 36–43.

Novak, Michael, *Free Persons and the Common Good* (New York: Madison Books, 1989).

Nozick, Robert, *Anarchy, State, and Utopia* (New York: Basic Books, 1971).

O'Donnell, John and James H. Taylor, "The Bounds of Charity," *The New England Journal of Medicine*, 322, no. 1 (Jan. 4, 1990): 65–68.

Olsen, E., "No Room at the Inn: A Snapshot of an American Emergency Room," *Stanford Law Review*, 46, no. 2 (Jan. 1994): 449–501.

Pelligrino, Edmund, "Compassion Needs Reason Too," *JAMA*, 270, no. 7, (Aug. 18, 1993): 874–5.

Pemberton, Prentiss, *Toward a Christian Economic Ethic: Stewardship and Social Power* (Minneapolis: Winston Press, 1985).

Pennock, J. Roland, and John W. Chapman, *Religion, Morality, and the Law* (New York: New York University Press, 1988).

Petrikin, Jonathan, *Male/Female Roles: Opposing Viewpoints* (San Diego, California: Greenhaven Press, 1995).

Peters, Tom, *In Search of Excellence* (New York: Harper and Row, 1982).

Plato, *The Collected Dialogues*, ed. by E. Hamilton and H. Cairns (Princeton, N.J.: Princeton University Press,

Povar, G. and J. Moreno, "Hippocrates and the Health Maintenance Organizations: A Discussion of Ethical Issues," *Annals of Internal Medicine*, 109, no. 5 (Sept. 1, 1988): 419–24.

Priester, Reinhard, "A Values Framework for Health System Reform," *Health Affairs*, 11, no. 1 (1992): 84–107.

Quill, Timothy, Christine Cassel and Diane Meier, "Care of the Hopelessly Ill: Proposed Guidelines for Physician-Assisted Suicide," *The New England Journal of Medicine*, 327, no. 19 (Nov. 5, 1992): 1380–1384.

Randall, James G. *Constitutional Problems Under Lincoln* (Urbana, Illinois: University of Illinois Press, 1964).

Raskin, Marcus, *The Common Good* (New York: Routledge and Kegan Paul, 1986).

Rawls, John, *A Theory of Justice* (Cambridge, Mass.: Harvard University Press 1971).

Reiman, Jeffrey, *In Defense of Political Philosophy*, (New York: Harper Torchbooks, 1972).

Relman, Arnold, "What Market Values are Doing to Medicine," *The Atlantic Monthly* (March 1992): 99–106.

Rennie, Drummond, Annette Flanagen, and Richard Glass, "Conflicts of Interest in the Publication of Science," *JAMA*, 226, no. 2 (July 10, 1991): 266–267.

Richardson, E. Allen, *Strangers in This Land: Pluralism and the Response to Diversity* (New York: Pilgrim Press, 1988).

Riker, William, *The Development of American Federalism* (Boston: Kluwer Academic Publishers, 1987).

Robertson, A. H., *Human Rights in Europe* (New York: Oceana Press, 1963).

Rodwin, Marc A., "Conflicts in Managed Care," *New England Journal of Medicine*, vol. 332, no. 9 (March 2, 1995): 604–607.

Rogot, E., P. Sorlie, N. Johnson, "Life Expectancy by Employment Status, Income, and Education in the National Longitudinal Mortality Study," *Public Health Reports*, 107, no. 4 (July 1992): 457–61.

Roth, John K., ed., *The Philosophy of Josiah Royce* (Indianapolis: Hackett Publishing Co., 1982).

Sade, Robert, "Medical Care as a Right: A Refutation," *The New England Journal of Medicine*, 285 (Dec. 2, 1971): 1288-1292.

Sartre, Jean-Paul, *Being and Nothingness*, trans. by Hazel Barnes (New York: Washington Square Press, 1966).

Satcher, D., "Should the Government Further Regulate Physician Supply? Yes." *Hospital Health Network*, 67, no. 17 (Sept. 5, 1993): 10.

Schnorr, Alvin L., "Job Turnover—A Problem with Employer-Based Health Care," *The New England Journal of Medicine*, 323, no. 8 (Aug. 23 1990): 543-545.

Seidman, Steven, *Embattled Eros: Sexual Politics and Ethics in Contemporary America* (New York: Routledge, 1992).

Shaw, K., S. Selbst, and F. Gill, "Indigent Children Who Are Denied Care in the Emergency Department," *Annals of Emergency Medicine*, 19, no. 1 (Jan. 1990): 59-62.

Sherover, Charles M., *Time, Freedom and the Common Good* (Albany: State University of New York Press, 1989).

Siddharthan K., and S. Alalasundaram, "Undocumented Aliens and Uncompensated Care: Whose Responsibility?" *American Journal of Public Health*, 83, no. 3 (March 1993): 410-12.

Siegler, Marc, "A Right to Health Care: Ambiguity, Professional Responsibility, and Patient Liberty," *Journal of Medicine and Philosophy*, 4, no. 2 (June 1979): 148-156.

Smart, J. C. C., and Bernard Williams, eds., *Utilitarianism, For and Against* (Cambridge: Cambridge University Press, 1973).

Smith, David, *With Willful Intent: A Theology of Sin* (Wheaton, Illinois: BridgePoint, 1993).

Solomon, Robert C., *Ethics and Excellence* (New York: Oxford University Press, 1992).

Sprung, C. and B. Winick, "Informed Consent in Theory and Practice," *Critical Care Medicine*, 17, no. 12 (Dec. 1989): 1346-54.

Starr, Paul, *The Social Transformation of American Medicine* (New York: Basic Books, 1982).

Stevens, Rosemary, *In Sickness and in Wealth: American Hospitals in the Twentieth Century* (New York: Basic Books, 1989).

Stone, V., J. Brown, and V. Sidel, "Decreasing the Field Strength of the National Health Service Corps: Will Access to Care Suffer?" *Journal of Health Care for the Poor and Underserved*, 2, no. 3 (Winter 1991): 347-58.

Swartz, Katherine, "Dynamics of People Without Health Insurance," *JAMA*, 271, no. 1 (January 5, 1994): 64-66.

——, *The Medically Uninsured*, (Washington D.C.: The Urban Institute, 1989).

Sykes, Charles J., *A Nation of Victims* (New York: St. Martin's Press, 1992).

Tancredi, L. and R. Bovbjerg, "Creating Outcomes-Based Systems for Quality and Malpractice Reform," *Milbank Quarterly*, 70, no. 1 (1992): 183-216.

Temkin, Owsei and Lilian Temkin, *Ancient Medicine* (Baltimore: Johns Hopkins Press, 1967).

Tingley, F., "A Use of Guidelines to Reduce Costs and Improve Quality: A Perspective from the Insurers," *Joint Commission Journal on Quality Improvement*, 19, no. 8 (Aug. 1993): 330-334.

Toner, Robin, "Groups Rally to Fight Medicare Cuts," *The New York Times*, (Dec. 18, 1994): 30.

Tronto, Joan C., *Moral Boundaries* (New York: Routledge, Chapman, and Hall, 1993).

Tucker, David M., *The Decline of Thrift in America*, (New York: Praeger, 1991).

Tyack, David, *Law and the Shaping of Public Education* (Madison, Wisconsin: University of Wisconsin Press, 1987).

United States General Accounting Office, "Long-Term Care: Other Countries Tighten Budgets While Seeking Better Access," (GAO/HEHS-94-154), Aug. 1994.

Vavala, D., "Medical Practices: Hot Properties of the 90s," *Physician Executive*, 19, no. 5 (Sept. 1993): 40-5.

Veatch, Robert, "What Counts as Basic Health Care? Private Values and Public Policy," *Hastings Center Report*, 24, no. 3 (May-June 1994).

Weiler, Paul, Joseph Newhouse, and Howard Hiatt, "Proposal for Medical Liability Reform," *JAMA*, 267, no. 17 (May 6, 1992): 2355-2358.

Wetzel, James, "American Families: 75 Years of Change," *Monthly Labor Review* (March 1990): 4-13.

"What the Taxman Takes," *The Economist* (March 13, 1993): 83-84.

White, Jane H., "ERISA May Hinder States As They Attempt Healthcare Reform," *Hospital Progress*, 75, no. 8 (Oct. 1994): 14-16.

———, "Health System Changes in the Absence of National Reform." *Health Progress*, 57, no. 10 (Dec. 1994): 10-12, 16.

Wills, Garry, *Explaining America: The Federalist* (Garden City, New York: Doubleday, 1981).

Wilson, James Q., *Bureaucracy: What Government Agencies Do and Why They Do It* (New York: Basic Books, 1989).

Wilson, S., and S. Walker, "Unemployment and Health: A Review," *Public Health*, 107, no. 3 (May 1993): 153-62.

Wise, Paul and DeWayne M. Pursey, "Infant Mortality as a Social Mirror," *The New England Journal of Medicine*, 326, no. 23 (June 4, 1992): 1558-1560.

Witt, Michael and Lawrence Gostin, "Conflict of Interest Dilemmas in Biomedical Research," *JAMA*, 271, no. 7 (Feb. 16, 1994): 547-551.

Wittgenstein, Ludwig, *Philosophical Investigations*, trans. by G. M. Anscombe (New York: Macmillan Company, 1968).

Wolff, Robert Paul, Barrington Moore, and Herbert Marcuse, *A Critique of Pure Tolerance* (Boston: Beacon Press, 1965).

Wolfe, Patricia and Donald Moran, "Global Budgeting in the OECD Countries," *Health Care Financing Review*, 14 no. 3 (Spring 1993): 55-76.

Woolhandler, Steffie and David Himmelstein, "The Deteriorating Administrative Efficiency of the U.S. Health Care System," *The New England Journal of Medicine*, 324, no. 18 (May 2, 1991): 1253-1257.

Wyszewianski, L., "Quality of Care: Past Achievements and Future Challenges," *Inquiry*, 25, no. 1 (Spring 1988): 13-22.

Index